Coping with Liver Disease

Mark Greener spent a decade in biomedical research before joining *MIMS Magazine* for GPs in 1989. Since then, he has written on health and biology for magazines worldwide for patients, healthcare professionals and scientists. He is the author of 13 other books, including *Coping with Asthma in Adults* (2011) and *The Heart Attack Survival Guide* (2012), both Sheldon Press. Mark lives with his wife, three children and two cats in a Cambridgeshire village.

Overcoming Common Problems Series

Selected titles

A full list of titles is available from Sheldon Press,
36 Causton Street, London SW1P 4ST and on our website at
www.sheldonpress.co.uk

101 Questions to Ask Your Doctor
Dr Tom Smith

Birth Over 35
Sheila Kitzinger

Coeliac Disease: What you need to know
Alex Gazzola

**Coping Successfully with Chronic Illness:
Your healing plan**
Neville Shone

Coping Successfully with Shyness
Margaret Oakes, Professor Robert Bor
and Dr Carina Eriksen

Coping with Anaemia
Dr Tom Smith

Coping with Asthma in Adults
Mark Greener

Coping with Bronchitis and Emphysema
Dr Tom Smith

Coping with Drug Problems in the Family
Lucy Jolin

Coping with Early-onset Dementia
Jill Eckersley

Coping with Eating Disorders and Body Image
Christine Craggs-Hinton

Coping with Gout
Christine Craggs-Hinton

**Coping with Manipulation: When others
blame you for their feelings**
Dr Windy Dryden

Coping with Obsessive Compulsive Disorder
Professor Kevin Gournay, Rachel Piper
and Professor Paul Rogers

Coping with Stomach Ulcers
Dr Tom Smith

Depressive Illness – the Curse of the Strong
Dr Tim Cantopher

The Diabetes Healing Diet
Mark Greener and Christine Craggs-Hinton

Dying for a Drink
Dr Tim Cantopher

**Epilepsy: Complementary and alternative
treatments**
Dr Sallie Baxendale

Fibromyalgia: Your Treatment Guide
Christine Craggs-Hinton

The Heart Attack Survival Guide
Mark Greener

How to Beat Worry and Stress
Dr David Delvin

How to Come Out of Your Comfort Zone
Dr Windy Dryden

How to Develop Inner Strength
Dr Windy Dryden

How to Eat Well When You Have Cancer
Jane Freeman

**Let's Stay Together: A guide to lasting
relationships**
Jane Butterworth

Living with IBS
Nuno Ferreira and David T. Gillanders

Losing a Parent
Fiona Marshall

**Making Sense of Trauma: How to tell
your story**
Dr Nigel C. Hunt and Dr Sue McHale

Motor Neurone Disease: A family affair
Dr David Oliver

Natural Treatments for Arthritis
Christine Craggs-Hinton

Overcoming Loneliness
Alice Muir

**The Pain Management Handbook:
Your personal guide**
Neville Shone

The Panic Workbook
Dr Carina Eriksen, Professor Robert Bor
and Margaret Oakes

Reducing Your Risk of Dementia
Dr Tom Smith

**Therapy for Beginners: How to get the best
out of counselling**
Professor Robert Bor, Sheila Gill
and Anne Stokes

**Transforming Eight Deadly Emotions
into Healthy Ones**
Dr Windy Dryden

Treating Arthritis: The drug-free way
Margaret Hills and Christine Horner

Treating Arthritis: The supplements guide
Julia Davies

**When Someone You Love Has Depression:
A handbook for family and friends**
Barbara Baker

Overcoming Common Problems

Coping with Liver Disease

MARK GREENER

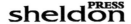

To Rory, Ophelia, Yasmin and Rose – with love

First published in Great Britain in 2013

Sheldon Press
36 Causton Street
London SW1P 4ST
www.sheldonpress.co.uk

British Library Cataloguing-in-Publication Data
A catalogue record for this book is available from the British Library

ISBN 978-1-84709-242-7
eBook ISBN 978-1-84709-243-4

Typeset by Fakenham Prepress Solutions, Fakenham, Norfolk NR21 8NN
First printed in Great Britain by Ashford Colour Press
Subsequently digitally printed in Great Britain

Produced on paper from sustainable forests

Contents

Note to the reader		vi
Introduction		vii
1	Inside a healthy liver	1
2	Symptoms of liver disease	11
3	Testing for liver disease	21
4	The A to E of viral hepatitis	28
5	Alcoholic liver disease	42
6	Non-alcoholic liver disease	52
7	Liver cancer	59
8	Other diseases of the liver	70
9	Diet and liver disease	82
10	Using herbs to cleanse the liver	99
11	Living with liver disease	113
Useful addresses		122
References		125
Further reading		132
Index		133

Note to the reader

This is not a medical book and is not intended to replace advice from your doctor. Consult your pharmacist or doctor if you believe you have any of the symptoms described, and if you think you might need medical help.

Introduction

Once upon a time, Greek legend tells, Zeus punished humanity by making us forget how to use fire. However, Prometheus restored our knowledge. In revenge, Zeus chained Prometheus to a rock and condemned the Titan to endure the torment of an eagle eating his liver for eternity. Prometheus's liver regenerated overnight, allowing the bird of prey to feast afresh the next day. Prometheus's torment lasted 13 generations until Herakles (the hero that the Romans adopted as Hercules) slew the eagle.[1]

Remarkably, the legend of Prometheus contains a kernel of truth: the liver's superlative powers of rejuvenation. Ancient Greeks possibly noted the organ's recuperative powers by observing wounds, while draining pus-filled abscesses, or when they used livers, often from sacrificed sheep and poultry, to try to divine the future.[1] This amazing ability to regenerate means that the liver recovers from injury and disease in a way few other human tissues can match. Indeed, the liver can regain its normal size and function even if a surgeon removes three-quarters of the organ.

Nevertheless, numerous diseases and unhealthy lifestyles can overwhelm the liver's legendary ability to recover. Indeed, liver disease kills approximately 1 in 50 people in the UK, according to a 2012 report from the National End of Life Care Intelligence Network. Sixty per cent of people who die from liver disease are men. And 90 per cent of people who die from liver disease are younger than 70 years of age. To make matters worse, the death toll is rising: from 9,231 in 2001 to 11,575 in 2009. Indeed, a 2011 report, *Making alcohol a health priority: Opportunities to reduce alcohol harms and rising costs,* from Alcohol Concern warned that liver disease could overtake strokes and heart disease as a cause of death within 10 to 20 years.

On the other hand, deaths from liver disease have fallen dramatically in some continental European countries in recent years. A study published in the *Lancet* estimated that reducing deaths from liver disease in the UK to the same extent as in France (the European Union country with the most profound decline in mortality) would save 22,000 lives by 2019. Even reaching the average reduction across Europe would save 8,900 lives over the same time.[2]

As you might expect from the sobering stories that regularly hit the headlines, alcohol abuse underlies much of the increasing death toll from liver disease. Indeed, epidemiologists (scientists who study patterns of disease) estimate that alcohol causes around 80 per cent of deaths from liver disease.[2] And according to the *British Journal of Cancer*, alcohol causes around 1 in every 25 cancers,[3] including malignancies in the liver, which, as we will see later in the book, carry a particularly bleak prognosis.

However, alcohol abuse is not the only cause of liver (hepatic) disease. Apart from causing lung cancer, smoking seems to promote malignancies in the liver. Viruses, diet, diabetes, autoimmune diseases (where the immune system's 'attack force' targets healthy tissue) and even wearing tight underwear can damage this critical organ. And the more liver diseases you have, the worse your prospects become. For example, the outlook for a person infected with a hepatitis virus is worse if they also drink excessively.

A silent killer

Occasionally, liver disease causes startling changes. For example, the liver makes haem – the red pigment in blood. Abnormal haem production can lead to the body excreting large amounts of proteins (called porphyrins), some of which can tinge urine red or purple. It's a startling and worrying symptom.

Usually, however, liver diseases do not cause dramatic symptoms – at least at first. For example, many people don't realize anything's amiss when they catch a hepatitis virus. Others dismiss the mild early symptoms as a bout of flu. But the virus lurks in your liver cells, flaring up years later to scar the liver (cirrhosis), cause jaundice or uncontrolled bleeding and, in some people, trigger hepatic cancer. Liver diseases can be silent killers.

The scourge of alcohol abuse aside, liver disease rarely attracts the same attention as heart conditions, dementia or breast cancer. However, as we will see over the course of this book, liver disease is common, can cause debilitating symptoms and may prove fatal. The course of each condition varies from person to person. In general, however, liver diseases progress from hepatitis (liver inflammation) to cirrhosis and cancer. As this progression typically takes 20–40 years,[4] you can often prevent, or at least delay, serious health problems.

Coming to terms with a doctor telling you that you have chronic (long-lasting) liver disease is rarely easy – especially as some hepatic conditions carry an unfavourable outlook or retain an unwarranted stigma. Too many people still think that cirrhosis inevitably means you're an alcoholic, or that catching a hepatitis virus means that you inject drugs or are sexually promiscuous, for example. But you don't need to feel that the ailment chains you to a rock, the disease pecking away at the remnants of your healthy liver.

This book aims to help you understand, treat and prevent liver disease. We will:

- review the liver's many roles (it is far more than a waste disposal system);
- examine the liver's often underestimated importance for our good health and well-being;
- look at the common liver diseases and their treatments;
- discuss some steps you can take to prevent liver disease, including a sensible approach to detox;
- look at the lifestyle changes that help you live as full and fulfilled a life as possible;
- consider which herbs offer effective 'liver tonics' and which can damage the organ.

The book aims to help you understand your liver disease and appreciate the best way to manage your symptoms, reduce the risk to your family and friends, and improve your prospects. I hope that, as well as resolving some immediate issues, this book will inspire further questions, which your doctor, nurse and pharmacist will be happy to answer. An active, enquiring approach helps you loosen the shackles of liver disease.

A word to the wise

This book does not replace advice from your liver specialist, GP or nurse, who will offer suggestions, support and treatment tailored to your circumstances. You should always see a doctor or nurse if you feel unwell or think that your liver disease is getting worse.

The book includes numerous references from medical and scientific studies. But it's been impossible to cite all those I referred to while writing the book. As you can imagine, researchers publish thousands of papers every year on liver disease (apologies to any researchers whose work I've missed). However, throughout the book I've highlighted certain papers to illustrate key points and themes.

If you want to know more about a study, I've given the reference in the back of the book. Some may seem rather erudite if you don't have a medical or biological background. But don't be put off. You can find a summary by entering the details here: <www.ncbi.nlm.nih.gov/pubmed>. Some full papers are available free online and larger libraries might also stock or allow you to access online some of the better-known medical journals.

1

Inside a healthy liver

Traditional healers have long regarded the liver as essential for health and well-being. For example, the liver is one of the five organs around which traditional Chinese medicine is organized. Jennifer Harper notes that, according to traditional Chinese medicine, the liver is home to the spiritual soul – called the *Hun*. And, writing around AD 200, the great Greco-Roman physician Galen suggested that the liver was the body's most important organ.[1] Yet, a couple of millennia later, the liver is arguably less well understood by the public than, for example, the heart, brain or lungs.

This chapter looks at the structure and roles of this vital organ. Parts may seem a little technical at first and you may need to read some sections again. You can also ask your doctor, nurse or a helpline if you're still unclear. (I've listed some useful addresses at the end of the book.) It's worth making the effort: this chapter will help you understand why certain liver diseases arise, allow you to appreciate why hepatic conditions can prove so devastating and to recognize the importance of ensuring you keep your liver healthy.

Inside your liver

Around the third week after conception, a small bud forms from the developing embryo's duodenum – the part of the gut just below the stomach. This bud develops into the liver and gall bladder. By the time you're an adult, a liver typically weighs between 1200 and 1500 g and is, apart from your skin, your body's largest organ.[2]

Occasionally, the liver buds that form during the embryo's development 'seed' in the wrong place. This results in small nodules of normal liver tissue near, for example, the kidneys, gall bladder and in the thorax. While less than 1 per cent of people show these 'ectopic' liver deposits, the nodules occasionally turn cancerous (Chapter 7).[2]

The gall bladder

A healthy gall bladder – a pear-shaped pouch under the liver, which is between 7 and 9 cm long – fills with and then concentrates bile, a greenish-yellow fluid produced by the liver. The gall bladder usually stores around 50 ml of bile – about 10 teaspoons worth. The gall bladder contracts when you eat. This pushes bile along tubes called ducts and into the duodenum.[2] Once in the duodenum, bile helps you digest fats in your diet.

Structure of the liver

A normal, healthy liver consists of two main lobes: the right lobe is about six times larger than the left. Doctors further divide the right lobe into the caudate and quadrate lobes.[2] (Many anatomical systems further subdivide the liver, but these don't need to concern us here.) The livers of several animals (such as pigs, dogs and camels) have more lobes than humans. Rarely, human livers also show additional lobes – up to 16 in some people – which are usually small and do not seem to cause health problems.[2]

Finding your liver

So where is your liver? Place your right hand over the lower right-hand side of your ribs. Your handprint roughly covers your liver (Figure 1.1). To be a little more accurate, the upper edge of the right lobe of your liver is level with your fifth rib (counted down from your shoulder), about 1 cm below your right nipple. The upper edge of the liver's left lobe is level with your sixth rib, about 2 cm below your left nipple.

On the left side of your body, the diaphragm (a thick muscular sheet that helps breathing) separates the liver from the bottom of the heart.[2] When you breathe in, the diaphragm flattens, pushing down on the liver. The diaphragm's movement can mean that the liver's edge falls by about 1–3 cm when you take a deep breath. A low diaphragm – for instance, in emphysema (page 75) – or when you take a *very* deep breath (such as those made by athletes or singers) can push the liver down even further. Indeed, severe, chronic (the technical term for long-lasting or persistent) cough can carve between one and six vertical furrows on the liver.[2]

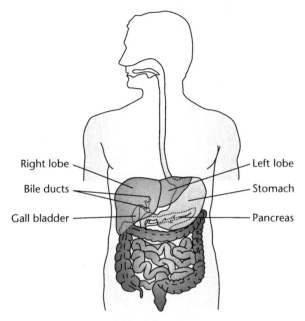

Figure 1.1 The position of a healthy liver

Through the microscope

If you look down a microscope at a slice of human liver, you will see rows of cells radiating from a central vein.[2] These cells – called hepatocytes – are the liver's main workhorse and make up about 60 per cent of the organ. Each hepatocyte is approximately 30–50 μm in diameter. A μm is one-millionth of a metre, so you could fit two or three hepatocytes across the thickness of an average piece of paper. One gram of normal liver contains approximately 2 million cells. Each liver cell lives for about 150 days.[2]

Looking at the liver through the microscope reveals several other types of cell. For example, Kupffer cells (a type of white blood cell) remove old and damaged blood cells, debris, bacteria, viruses, parasites and cancer cells. Alcohol undermines the Kupffer cells' ability to remove this debris and potentially harmful micro-organisms.[2] That is just one of many reasons why alcohol causes liver damage (Chapter 5).

The body's waste disposal unit

The liver's ability to remove waste is probably the organ's best-known role, although as we'll see, waste disposal is far from being the only hepatic function.

When you eat, food passes along your food pipe (oesophagus), through your stomach and into your gut (gastrointestinal tract). Obviously, humans did not always get their food fresh, analysed for quality and wrapped in cellophane on regularly cleaned shop shelves. Often, our ancestors ate food scavenged or collected in the wild, sometimes decaying or caked in dirt. Water came from rivers and ponds – not filtered and purified from the taps.

So, we inevitably ingested natural poisons, microbes and other chemicals along with our food and drink. As Andrew Weil notes, black peppers, basil, tarragon, alfalfa sprouts, celery, peanuts, potatoes, tomatoes and white mushrooms potentially contain toxins. (Unfortunately, this list includes many of my favourite foods.) But, as we'll see when we look at aflatoxin (page 61), you usually need to eat large amounts for a long time to experience any harmful effects – partly because levels of the toxin are so low and partly because your body has evolved formidable defences.

These natural poisons, microbes and other chemicals enter the dense network of blood vessels that supplies the gut. In turn, most of the blood supply from your gut passes through the liver before reaching the rest of the body. This allows your liver to filter blood, and detect and destroy many potentially harmful chemicals and microorganisms before they can damage the rest of the body. (The technical term for this is first-pass metabolism.)

The rich blood supply from the rest of the body allows the liver to remove harmful by-products of the chemical processes that keep us alive, as well as chemicals that eluded first-pass metabolism. For example, the liver removes about 1 unit of alcohol from your blood every hour, although people differ dramatically in the speed at which they metabolize alcohol.

The liver also receives and filters lymph, a clear, yellowish fluid that bathes our tissues and contains white blood cells, which help you fight off infections. As a result, your lymph nodes (such as the 'glands' under your chin and in your armpits) may swell when you have an infection. Lymph circulates through the network of vessels called the lymphatic system, collecting unwanted materials for removal by, for example, the liver.

A colourful process

In many cases, enzymes in the liver break down chemicals to less harmful 'metabolites' that the body can remove more easily, usually either in bile (and, in turn, the faeces) and urine. An enzyme is a specialized protein that ensures a chemical reaction in the body works effectively and efficiently. Without enzymes, many biological reactions would not take place quickly enough to ensure we stay healthy.

For example, the liver may convert a chemical into a metabolite that dissolves in water more readily. This helps your kidneys expel the metabolite in your urine. One large group of enzymes is especially important: the cytochrome P450 system (see box 'The cytochromes'). Indeed, the cytochrome P450 system breaks down about three-quarters of medicines, which may mean doctors need to be careful which drugs they prescribe to people with liver disease (see 'The risk of drug interactions' elsewhere in this chapter and see also page 79).[3]

However, the cytochrome P450 system and other metabolic enzymes may not inactivate all chemicals. Indeed, the liver converts some inactive chemicals, including certain medicines, into

The cytochromes

The term 'cytochrome' refers to coloured (the ancient Greek word for colour is *chrome*), iron-containing proteins in cells (the ancient Greek word for cell is *cyto*). Each of the colours in a rainbow represents a particular wavelength of light. Certain biological proteins appear coloured because they absorb a particular wavelength of light. For example, a wavelength of 450 nm is roughly equivalent to the boundary between blue and violet visible light. One group of metabolic enzymes found in several places in the body, but particularly in the liver, absorbs light at 450 nm. So, biochemists named this enzyme group cytochrome P450 (the 'P' refers to pigment). Other iron-containing proteins, such as haemoglobin in blood, absorb a different wavelength, which is why blood appears red.

an active form called a reactive or active metabolite. The liver may attach another chemical to help inactivate and excrete these active metabolites.

The liver produces numerous specialized metabolic enzymes to allow us to contend with the wide range of potentially hazardous chemicals we encounter every day. Indeed, the liver can fine-tune production of these enzymes to meet particular hazards. For example, levels of a certain liver enzyme (gamma-glutamyltrans-ferase) increase in around three-quarters of chronic drinkers. So, doctors measure certain key enzymes (page 24) to help determine our liver's health.

The risk of drug interactions

Some medicines trigger the liver to increase production of a particular cytochrome P450 enzyme – so-called inducers. If you take the inducer with another medicine broken down by same enzyme, the liver may remove the second drug more quickly. St John's wort (*Hypericum perforatum*), a widely used herbal antidepressant, potently induces one cytochrome, called CYP3A4. So, CYP3A4 levels rise if you take St John's wort. If you also take a medicine metabolized by CYP3A4, the higher level of this enzyme rapidly breaks the medicine down and the drug may not work as well as it should (page 79).

On the other hand, several drugs and herbs – and even grapefruit juice – inhibit CYP3A4. Taking a drug metabolized by CYP3A4 along with a medicine that inhibits the same enzyme allows the blood level of the first medicine to rise, which could cause side effects. This risk of interactions is one reason why you should let your doctor and pharmacist know when you are using herbal remedies (page 103) and other medicines bought over the counter.

However, liver cells that break down potential toxins inevitably receive a greater dose of potentially harmful chemicals than other hepatocytes. And because they need to remove the poisons, these cells lack some of the defences that other hepatocytes use to limit damage. So, these essential cells are particularly susceptible to chemicals that can damage the liver, such as paracetamol (page 81) and carbon tetrachloride, once used in some fire extinguishers and dry cleaning fluid.[2] Liver damage from other causes (such as viruses, excess fat and alcohol) can reduce the organ's ability to deal with these dangerous chemicals. So, people with liver disease need to avoid, as far as possible, any medicines or other chemicals that can damage hepatic cells.

Supplying our energy demands

Traditionally, people ate a plate of liver and onions to give themselves a boost. Apart from containing large amounts of iron, the liver is rich in easily used sources of energy.

The body can use several fuels, although glucose is the most common. We usually obtain glucose by breaking down starch and sugars in food. As blood from the gut flows through the organ, liver cells remove between 25 and 30 per cent of the glucose absorbed from the meal. The liver uses about 60 per cent of this glucose to fuel its activities. Liver cells stick the rest of the glucose together into a long chain called glycogen, which is a bit like a biological battery. Glycogen stores energy ready for future use, when, for example, you're more active or you haven't eaten for several hours. When you wake in the morning, your liver has produced about 80 per cent of the glucose circulating in your blood. Your kidneys have released the other 20 per cent. After a meal, levels of glucose in the blood rise. In response, the amount of glucose released from the liver declines by almost 80 per cent.[4]

Stockpiles of glycogen in the liver and muscle store about 2,000 calories worth of energy in a 70 kg person. A moderately active person needs about 16 calories a day for each pound of body weight to keep their weight stable. Sedentary people and those who exercise vigorously need about 13 and 18 calories, respectively, for each pound of body weight. In other words, the glycogen stores are enough to keep an average woman going for a day.

Production declines dramatically once glycogen stores make up more than about 5 per cent of the liver's weight. But glucose is too valuable to waste. Our ancestors often – literally – did not know where their next meal was coming from. So, liver cells convert the additional glucose into other chemicals called fatty acids. The liver releases fatty acids into the circulation.

Triglycerides and liver disease

Several tissues use fatty acids as a fuel when there is not enough glucose. In times of plenty, however, fat cells (adipocytes) take up glucose, which they use to make another chemical called glycerol. Adipocytes then join glycerol to the fatty acids produced by the liver to form fats called triglycerides – yet another energy store.

Cholesterol and triglycerides are both fats. However, they have very different biological roles (we'll look at the role of the much maligned cholesterol later in the chapter.) When you eat, your body 'burns' carbohydrates (such as sugar) to meet your immediate energy needs. The body converts any leftover calories into triglycerides, which you store in fat cells. You can then use the energy later. But as we tend to eat regularly, we rarely use these energy stores. So, we keep piling on the pounds. The body of a 70 kg adult stores around 100,000 calories as triglycerides, mostly in layers of fat – especially around the stomach. That's one reason why a bulging waistline (central obesity) increases the likelihood of developing several conditions, including heart disease, certain cancers and fatty liver disease (page 52). As we'll see in Chapter 6, a healthy liver contains very little fat.

Finally, the liver contributes to yet another mechanism that helps us survive food shortages. And you can see its effects by looking at those tragic pictures of famine victims or people with anorexia, who seem little more than skin and bones. When we've depleted our other energy stores, cells start breaking down muscle. This releases the building blocks of protein (amino acids) into the bloodstream. The liver can convert some amino acids into glucose – a process called gluconeogenesis. This 'starvation reaction' is one reason why it is better to lose weight slowly and steadily (page 94) rather than crash diet. Indeed, crash diets can be especially harmful to the liver.

Cholesterol: the misunderstood fat

The liver makes cholesterol,[2] which, despite its bad press, is an essential part of the membranes surrounding every cell and the insulation (myelin sheath) around many nerves that ensures that signals travel properly. And cholesterol forms the backbone of several hormones, including oestrogen, testosterone and progesterone. But poor diets and a lack of exercise (which burns up fat) mean that many of us have too much of a good thing.

Transporting cholesterol around the body poses a problem. Blood is about four-fifths water. As oil and water do not mix, your body surrounds a core of cholesterol with soluble coats called lipoproteins, including:

- Low-density lipoprotein (LDL) carries cholesterol from the liver to the tissues. LDL accumulates in artery walls, forming the fatty deposits (called plaques) that cause most heart attacks and contribute to strokes, kidney damage and some other diseases.
- High-density lipoprotein (HDL) carries cholesterol from the arteries to the liver for excretion.

In other words, high LDL levels increase the risk of heart attacks and other diseases. High levels of HDL protect against these conditions. It's easy to remember: LDL is 'lethal'; HDL is 'healthy'.

The liver's other actions

The liver has several other roles that are critical for health and well-being, including:

- Galen regarded the liver as the main site of blood production.[1] Today, we know that the bone marrow makes almost all the blood flowing around an adult's body. However, the liver produces most of the blood in a developing embryo, starting around the 12th week following conception. Bone marrow does not take over until the fifth month of pregnancy. In adults, the liver still makes haem: part of haemoglobin, the molecule that carries oxygen in red blood cells.[2] As we'll see, porphyria (page 70) arises from defects in the haem production line.
- Vitamin A is important for vision, healthy bones, reproduction and an effective immune system. The liver stores between 22 and 220 days' worth of vitamin A.[5]
- The liver produces about 9–12 g of a protein called albumin each day. Albumin helps maintain the delicate balance between the amount of fluid in your blood and your tissues. Albumin also transports calcium, several hormones (including testosterone and progesterone) and numerous medicines to their site of action.

- When you cut yourself, a complicated series of proteins (the coagulation cascade) stems the flow of blood and starts repairing the damage. The liver produces an array of these proteins, which stop us bleeding to death, as well as those that prevent harmful and unnecessary clots forming inside the body. The liver also clears these coagulation factors from the bloodstream, again helping to prevent excessive clotting. Not surprisingly, some liver diseases can trigger bleeding problems.

The liver may not attract the same attention from poets as the heart, from scientists as the brain or from the public as the breast. However, the liver is at least as important to our health and well-being. The liver's central role in numerous critical biological processes helps explain why hepatic conditions can prove devastating, debilitating and even deadly. In Chapter 2, we'll look at some common symptoms that might suggest that you have liver disease.

2

Symptoms of liver disease

As the legend of Prometheus illustrates, the liver can compensate for even relatively extensive damage. As a result, symptoms often emerge only once hepatic disease is relatively advanced. Early on, you might be unaware that you're damaging your liver – and so you keep eating poorly, drinking excessively, smoking, or not tackling the viral infection. As a result, the damage continues. To complicate matters further, many symptoms caused by a poorly functioning liver are vague and easily confused with other diseases.

So, deciding based on symptoms alone whether you have liver disease, and if so which type, is often difficult. Indeed, many of the hallmark symptoms of liver disease we'll discuss in this chapter – such as a swollen, tender, inflamed liver (hepatitis), the yellow tinge of jaundice, a swollen stomach and scarring (cirrhosis) – can arise from very different triggers. Often if you remove the trigger (take antivirals, quit drinking and eat a healthy diet, for example) the liver can recover.

However, if exposure to the trigger continues, persistent (chronic) inflammation can lead to cirrhosis, end-stage liver disease and even cancer. But liver disease's slow development usually offers a window of opportunity to prevent further progression, often even if the damage is already relatively advanced. So, if you develop any of the symptoms in this chapter, or feel otherwise unwell, you should see your GP.

Jodie's story
Jodie, a 23-year-old team leader in a high-street fashion store, felt fatigued, depressed and anxious after she returned for travelling in Thailand. She lost her appetite and found she could not concentrate as well as she used to when she reconciled the day's takings. And her abdomen felt bloated and tender. Jodie put the symptoms down to her jet lag and changes in diet. However, she had contracted hepatitis C virus from a dirty needle used to give her a tattoo in Bangkok.

Table 2.1 Possible symptoms of liver disease

See your GP if you develop any of the following:
  Fatigue and weakness
  Feeling generally unwell
  Loss of appetite
  Nausea, vomiting or both
  Unexplained weight loss (e.g. without dieting)
  Pain or discomfort in the abdomen
  Feeling itchy, especially if severe
  Small red veins that look a bit like a spider (spider naevi)
  Enlarged and tender liver, especially below your right ribs
  Dark, brown urine
  Grey, pale, clay-coloured stools (faeces)
  Loss of sex drive
*See your GP **immediately** if you develop any of the following:*
  Yellow tinge to your skin and eyes (jaundice)
  Swollen abdomen
  Dark or black, tarry faeces
  Fever with high temperature and shivering
  Vomiting blood

Source: Adapted from the British Liver Trust

If you experience any symptom in the top part of Table 2.1 you should see your doctor, especially if you could have been exposed to any high-risk situations. The symptoms in the lower part of the table may indicate severe liver disease. So, you should see your doctor as soon as possible.

Cirrhosis

When you injure yourself, scars protect the vulnerable area while your body repairs the damage. When the damage is short-lived, hepatic scarring helps your liver return to normal. But, over time, repeated damage and inflammation can lead to more extensive scarring, known as fibrosis. Eventually, hard, irregular areas of scar tissue, called nodules, replace the smooth liver. As a result, the liver can feel harder. The nodules can also hinder the flow of blood, which can starve liver cells of the oxygen and nutrients they need to survive. This extensive scarring means that the liver does not work properly – a condition called cirrhosis.

The liver can compensate for early scarring and inflammation and, over time, provided you stop damaging your liver, mild fibrosis can resolve. Cirrhosis tends to emerge when the damage to the liver is long term and unrelenting, such as in people who drink excessively for many years. Indeed, the risk of developing cirrhosis doubles if you drink more than 50 g alcohol daily (about 6 units – see page 43) and increases approximately fivefold among those drinking more than 100 g a day.[1] However, several genetic and other factors influence your likelihood of developing cirrhosis. So, as we'll see in Chapter 5, even large amounts of alcohol do not inevitably cause cirrhosis. But even if you manage to avoid scarring your liver, the other health, social and legal consequences of alcohol abuse can be devastating.

While many people seem to equate cirrhosis with alcohol abuse, numerous other 'insults' can scar the liver. For example, around 1 in 10 to 1 in 4 people infected with hepatitis C virus (HCV) develop cirrhosis. HCV (page 35) can directly damage liver cells, causing fibrosis and cirrhosis. However, cirrhosis can also arise as the immune system tries to eradicate HCV, by attacking and destroying infected liver cells.

Symptoms of cirrhosis

As we've seen, damage that persists for many years can produce extensive scarring that irrevocably changes the liver's architecture and function. Symptoms of cirrhosis develop because the scarred tissue does not work properly. If you have or develop any of the symptoms in the Table 2.2, you should see your GP as soon as possible.

Itching and liver disease

People with chronic liver disease can suffer from severe itching (pruritus). In some cases, the itching affects one part of the body, such as the hands or feet. In other cases, the pruritus is more widespread. The itching seems to arise when the liver cannot remove toxins (such as bilirubin; see page 17), which then build up in the body. Many people find that moisturizers and oatmeal baths alleviate the itching. Your doctor may also be able to suggest antihistamines and other drugs that may relieve the discomfort.

Compensated and decompensated cirrhosis

Once cirrhosis develops, the liver cannot repair the damage. Nevertheless, removing the cause (such as alcohol abuse) often prevents cirrhosis from getting worse: the liver's spare capacity may

Table 2.2 Symptoms of cirrhosis

Tiredness
Weakness
Loss of appetite
Unexplained weight loss
Nausea
Severe itching (pruritus)
Tenderness or pain around your liver
Spider naevi above your waist
Jaundice*
Bleeding problems*
Hair loss
Fever and shivering (the liver damage means you are more likely to pick up a bug)
Oedema (accumulation of fluid in your legs, ankles and feet)
Ascites*

*See the relevant sections elsewhere in this chapter.
Source: Adapted from NHS Direct

allow the organ to compensate for early cirrhosis, often for many years. So, doctors divide cirrhosis into two types: compensated and decompensated. In compensated cirrhosis, the liver's spare capacity means that the organ can still perform many important tasks, often despite extensive scarring.

However, liver damage may not progress consistently and symptoms can suddenly take a turn for the worse. Scientists are making remarkable progress in understanding the factors that contribute to cirrhosis. But doctors cannot yet predict accurately who will develop cirrhosis and how the condition will progress. So, you will probably need regular monitoring.

In decompensated cirrhosis, the extensive scarring prevents the liver from working properly and, not surprisingly, can cause debilitating symptoms and potentially life-threatening complications (see below). For example, cirrhosis is a leading cause of portal hypertension. (Several other hepatic conditions also cause portal hypertension.) Indeed, over 5 years, up to one-fifth (14–20 per cent) of people with compensated cirrhosis due to chronic hepatitis B virus infection (page 30) die, rising to about three-quarters (70–80 per cent) with decompensated cirrhosis.[2]

Portal hypertension

The hepatic portal vein carries blood from your digestive tract and spleen to your liver. Your spleen, which is normally about the size of your fist, lies above your stomach and under your ribs on the left side of your body. The spleen, part of your lymphatic system (page 4), has several important roles including:

- storing white blood cells (which fight infection), red blood cells and platelets (which help blood clot);
- helping to control the amount of blood circulating around your body;
- destroying old and damaged blood cells;
- making red blood cells (in certain circumstances) and some white blood cells (although bone marrow produces most blood cells).

Portal hypertension means that the blood pressure is dangerously high in the hepatic portal vein. Portal hypertension can force blood along smaller vessels to find a way back to the heart, causing them to swell, which potentially forms varices (see below). This increased pressure may also mean that the spleen swells with blood. A spleen swollen by portal hypertension is less able to store red and white blood cells. It is also less able to store platelets, which is one reason why people with cirrhosis are particularly likely to experience bleeding problems (see below).

Osteoporosis

Depending on the people studied and way the scientists designed the investigation, between 10 and 60 per cent of people with liver cirrhosis develop osteoporosis (brittle bone disease), leaving them at risk of debilitating fractures. As we get older the skeleton's strength naturally declines (the decline is especially marked in post-menopausal women). But many factors potentially further weaken bones in people with cirrhosis, including muscle wasting (see below), alcoholism, hormonal changes (see below) and low levels of vitamin D.[3]

So, everyone should make sure they consume sufficient vitamin D, especially if they don't spend very long outside (the skin makes vitamin D from sunlight.) A recent study of people aged 65 years or more found that taking between 792 and 2,000 IU vitamin D a day reduced the risk of hip and all non-spinal fractures by 30 per cent and 14 per cent, respectively.[4] You might need a vitamin D supplement (speak to your doctor if you have liver disease or any other health problem) to reach this level.

Increasing the amount of fish you eat will also help. The amount of vitamin D in 75 g of swordfish, salmon or canned tuna is around 570, 450 and 150 IU, respectively. As we'll see on page 88, fish is an excellent source of other essential nutrients that may help liver disease.

Mental changes

People with chronic liver disease can experience a range of mental problems. Some problems, such as depression and anxiety, may arise from the burden imposed by living with a serious disease and as a side effect of some treatments (page 37). In other cases, the liver disease directly causes the mental distress.

Cirrhosis, for example, can lead to mental problems including personality changes, altered sleep patterns, violent behaviour, sluggish movements, speech problems, drowsiness, confusion and poor mental performance, stupor, and coma. These changes (called hepatic encephalopathy) seem to arise from a combination of inflammation spilling out from the liver into the body, as well as high levels of ammonia and other toxins that healthy hepatocytes usually filter from the blood. The toxins and inflammation can cause certain nerve and other cells in the brain to swell. Meanwhile, the amount of fluid in the brain increases (cerebral oedema).[5]

You should see your doctor if you experience mental changes (including depression or anxiety – see page 117). If you have hepatic encephalopathy, your doctor may prescribe a laxative (such as lactulose), which may help remove toxins from the body. That's another good reason to eat a high-fibre diet (page 90) to ensure regular bowel movements. Furthermore, many cases of hepatic encephalopathy follow infections, constipation, dehydration, bleeding or treatment with certain medicines. So, your doctor will try to identify and treat any underlying cause.

Other complications

Scarring to the liver can cause numerous other complications, including:

Muscle wasting As the liver cannot process proteins effectively, a person with cirrhosis can lose muscle. So, they feel physically weak and are more likely to fracture a bone.

Hormonal changes The liver helps regulate the production and breakdown of some female and male hormones. So, cirrhosis can change hormone levels causing, for example, irregular menstrual periods in women and gynaecomastia (breast enlargement) in men. Hormonal changes may also weaken the skeleton, contributing to osteoporosis.

Kidney disease Some people with decompensated cirrhosis show worsening kidney (renal) function. As the kidneys remove excess fluid from the body, renal disease can contribute to fluid retention, which can in turn result in ascites (see below) and oedema (swelling) in the feet and legs. The increased strain on the renal system can promote kidney disorders. Kidney failure in people with cirrhosis is called hepatorenal syndrome.

Bleeding problems As we mentioned in Chapter 1, the liver produces chemicals that help your blood clot properly. So, a liver damaged by cirrhosis (especially once decompensated) may not produce sufficient clotting factors. To make matters worse, release of platelets from a spleen enlarged by portal hypertension may decline. As a result, many people with cirrhosis find that they tend to bleed and bruise more easily and have, for example, frequent nosebleeds or bleeding gums. To keep an eye on this problem, your doctor may regularly measure how quickly your blood clots.

Jaundice

Patients with jaundice – from the French for yellow (*jaune*) – develop a yellow tinge to their skin and whites of their eyes. The spleen (page 15) destroys old and damaged red blood cells. The breakdown of haemoglobin releases a yellowish product called bilirubin. The liver excretes most of the released bilirubin in bile, which flows into the intestine. Faeces' brown colour comes from the conversion of bilirubin into another chemical called stercobilin in the gut. You expel the rest of the bilirubin in your urine after conversion into urobilin – a yellowish pigment.

Several liver ailments trigger a rise in bilirubin in the bloodstream, potentially triggering jaundice. For instance, liver cancer can spread into and block bile ducts. So, bile cannot drain away. In other cases, hepatitis viruses, drugs, alcohol, cirrhosis and so on kill liver cells. So, the liver cannot process bilirubin for excretion.

As levels of bile and bilirubin in the blood rise, the kidneys excrete more bilirubin and there is less in the faeces. As a result, urine can turn dark brown. The faeces become pale and clay-coloured.

You should always make sure that your doctor uncovers the cause of your jaundice. For example, around one-quarter of people who go to their GP with jaundice have undiagnosed cancer. Researchers looked at the medical records of 277 men and women in the UK aged more than 45 years with jaundice. One-third (33 per cent) had bile duct stones (page 77), while 27 per cent had a malignancy that could account for the jaundice, including pancreatic cancer (12 per cent) and cholangiocarcinoma (5 per cent), a malignancy in the bile duct. Excess alcohol consumption accounted for 9 per cent of cases and 'other diagnoses' for another 9 per cent.[6]

Worryingly, more than 1 in 5 (22 per cent) records did not include a diagnosis that could explain the jaundice. However, many patients with jaundice have a serious disease, which highlights the importance of urgent investigations, including blood tests for, for example, viral hepatitis or autoimmune liver disease, and ultrasound scans to identify cancer and some other diseases.[6] So, if you develop jaundice see your doctor as soon as possible and insist on further tests.

Ascites

Liver disease and certain cancers cause fluid to build up between the tissues lining the abdomen and the organs – called ascites. Around three-quarters of ascites develop when cirrhosis squeezes blood vessels inside the liver. So, blood begins to back up. The increasing pressure forces blood from the vessels into the abdomen. Indeed, the accumulation of fluid can leave the person looking heavily pregnant. Apart from being unsightly and uncomfortable, ascites may press on the diaphragm. As a result, the lungs cannot expand fully, leaving you short of breath.

An ultrasound scan can detect ascites when 500 ml of fluid (in some cases less) collects in the abdomen. However, you'll usually notice the difference (and doctors can detect the build-up without resorting to imaging) once about 1500 ml of fluid has accumulated. Less fluid can make a noticeable difference in thinner people. Similarly, much more fluid needs to accumulate before ascites emerge in obese people.

Around half of people with cirrhosis develop ascites over a decade. Cancers – not just of the liver but also several others tumours, including those in the stomach, colon, ovary and pancreas – cause around 15 per cent of ascites. A variety of less common conditions causes the remaining cases.

If you develop ascites, doctors may advise that you reduce the amount of salt (which causes the body to retain water) you eat. Indeed, most people eat too much salt, whether or not they have liver disease. We'll look at ways to reduce your salt consumption in Chapter 9. Doctors may also prescribe diuretics (water tablets). These drugs make you excrete more dilute urine, reducing the amount of fluid in your body. In some cases, a surgeon may drain fluid from your abdomen.

Varices

Around 60 per cent of people with cirrhosis show varices,[7] which develop when portal hypertension stretches the veins supplying the upper part of stomach, the lower food pipe (oesophagus) and rectum. (The veins swell as blood tries to bypass the liver and get back to the heart.) In severe cases, swollen veins protrude into the oesophagus, forming varices.

Many of these blood vessels never evolved to resist this level of pressure: their walls are not thick enough. So, some varices slowly leak blood, possibly causing anaemia, which you may experience as, for example, tiredness, lack of energy and shortness of breath. Varices can also burst, causing severe bleeding (haemorrhage) and you may vomit blood or pass stools streaked with black blood.

Such problems are relatively common. Between 40 and 45 per cent of patients with large varices due to cirrhosis experience at least one bleed a year. And up to half of people who develop bleeding varices die.[7] So, *you must go to accident and emergency or call an ambulance if you or someone you know vomits blood. You should see your doctor urgently if you start passing bloody faeces.* Apart from liver disease, blood in your stools can be a sign of other diseases, including colon cancer.

Treating varices

Varices can be treated in several ways:

- By placing a small band around the varices to stop the bleeding.
- By injecting a chemical into the varices to trigger clotting and

scarring. This approach (called sclerotherapy) closes the vessel, preventing further bleeding.

- By passing a tube with a balloon on the end into the stomach. When inflated, the balloon squeezes the varices, which helps reduce bleeding.
- If these approaches do not control the bleeding, the swollen vessel can be bypassed by joining two larger veins with a metal tube called a stent. This reduces the pressure in the varices.
- You may also need to take drugs to reduce your blood pressure (antihypertensives). One group of antihypertensives – called beta-blockers – roughly halves the risk that varices will bleed.[7]

End-stage liver disease

Eventually, the liver damage can mean that the organ can no longer perform its normal functions; a condition called end-stage liver disease. Not surprisingly, people with end-stage liver disease develop serious symptoms. Doctors try to manage complications caused by a deteriorating liver. However, a liver transplant is the only effective treatment.

According to the NHS, between 600 and 700 people receive liver transplants each year in the UK. However, the lack of donated organs means that each year hundreds of people die who could have lived if they had received a transplant. Some people donate part of their liver while they are still alive (so-called living donation) to save the life of a relative or friend. As mentioned in the introduction, the healthy liver can regenerate.

Surgeons performed the world's first liver transplant in 1963 in Denver, Colorado. A team at Addenbrooke's Hospital in Cambridge performed the UK's first liver transplant 5 years later. Liver transplants have saved countless lives since these pioneering operations. But even if you receive a transplanted organ from a friend or family member it is still foreign to your body. This means that your immune system may try to attack the transplant, a process called rejection. So, you'll need to take immunosuppressant drugs. As these inhibit the immune system, using immunosuppressant drugs long term can cause side effects, including making you more likely to contract infections with viruses, bacteria, fungi and parasites, and increasing your risk of developing skin cancer and some other malignancies. Nevertheless, the benefits usually far outweigh the risks. Transplants are a true medical miracle.

3

Testing for liver disease

Liver diseases often produce rather vague symptoms. Indeed, many people with early liver disease do not develop any symptoms. To complicate matters further, several different conditions can cause the same symptom. So, doctors use a variety of tests to determine whether you have a particular liver disease, assess your likely progression and track your response to treatment. Each test has advantages and disadvantages, and offers a different view of your liver's health.

Virology and immunology

Several viruses can cause hepatitis (Chapter 4). So, doctors may take a blood sample to determine whether an infection might cause your symptoms and, if so, which virus you've caught. In some cases, doctors measure molecules produced by the virus – such as RNA, which is part of the virus's genetic machinery. In other cases, doctors measure levels of the antibodies made by your body to fight the virus.

Doctors may also regularly measure levels of the virus in your blood – the viral load – to see how well you are responding to treatment. For example, doctors regard people who have undetectable levels of HCV 24 weeks after the end of treatment as showing a sustained virological response. In other words, treatment may have cured the infection. But because the test cannot detect very low levels of the virus, doctors cannot yet be certain the infection is gone. As we'll see in Chapter 4, some viruses that cause hepatitis consist of a range of subtypes, which differ in their susceptibility to certain treatments. Virological testing allows doctors to decide on the most effective treatment for your infection.

Autoimmune diseases

Usually, antibodies detect and help white blood cells destroy invading bacteria, viruses (including those that cause hepatitis) and parasites, as well as mopping up potentially cancerous cells. However, occasionally, antibodies attack healthy cells.

Antibodies that attack the joints can cause rheumatoid arthritis. When antibodies attack the fatty sheath that surrounds some nerves – rather like plastic insulation surrounding a wire – patients can develop multiple sclerosis. During primary biliary cirrhosis, an autoimmune attack slowly destroys the bile ducts (Chapter 8). Autoimmune hepatitis follows an attack on the liver cells by the body's immune system.

Furthermore, the inflammation caused by several autoimmune diseases – including type 1 diabetes (the type that usually emerges in childhood), ulcerative colitis (autoimmune damage to the large intestine) and rheumatoid arthritis – can spill over and inflame the liver. So, doctors may measure levels of autoantibodies to see whether autoimmune reactions cause or contribute to your liver disease.

Imaging

In 1895, the German scientist Wilhelm Conrad Röentgen accidently discovered X-rays while experimenting with vacuum tubes. A week later, Röentgen took the first radiograph: of his wife's hand. The X-ray clearly showed her bones and wedding ring. Bones and teeth are denser, and so absorb more X-rays, than other tissues. The X-ray film or, more commonly today, detectors show bones as silhouettes.

Angiography

Unfortunately, soft organs such as the liver are not dense enough to reveal sufficient detail on X-rays to help doctors. So, during a process called angiography, the radiographer injects a 'contrast medium' into your blood vessels using a catheter (a thin, flexible, hollow tube). The contrast medium absorbs X-rays and, therefore, outlines the blood vessels. The X-ray (angiogram) then shows the site and severity of changes in blood flow through the liver. The angiogram may localize abnormalities, including tumours, in the liver and help surgeons plan operations.

Ultrasonography

During an ultrasound scan, a detector picks up sound waves as they bounce off tissue, building up a detailed picture of, for example, your liver, bile duct and gall bladder. The principle is the same as the prenatal scans used during pregnancy. Ultrasonography can detect changes in the liver's size and shape as well as revealing fatty deposits (steatosis) as bright white areas. However, steatosis usually needs to affect more than 30 per cent of the liver before an ultrasound scan can detect the fat deposits.[1] Furthermore, ultrasonography may not detect fibrosis.

CT and MRI

CT (computed tomography; sometimes called CAT – computerized axial tomography) and MRI (magnetic resonance imaging) scans visualize the inside of your body in often awe-inspiring detail. For example, CT uses X-rays to produce numerous (often more than a hundred) 'slices' through your tissue and organs. The beam varies in width, depending on the detail needed, from 1 mm to 10 mm. A computer rebuilds the slices into a single three-dimensional image in remarkably high resolution. In some cases, radiologists use a contrast medium to enhance the fine detail. MRI uses powerful magnetic fields to provide an even more detailed view than CT. Both CT and MRI can detect tumours, help detect the cause of jaundice, guide biopsies and so on.

But when you look at an organ in unprecedented detail, you're also more likely to detect previously unrecognized abnormalities. For instance, detailed scans have shown 'corset liver' in some elderly women who wore excessively tight underwear for many years. The pressure from their underwear produced a horizontal scar on the liver's usually glass-smooth surface. Similarly, imaging has shown that some people have Riedel's lobe, a tongue-like growth from the liver's right lobe. Riedel's lobe does not cause symptoms and does not need treatment.[2]

The risks and benefits of liver biopsy

Despite the remarkable advances in imaging, a liver biopsy may be the only way to confirm that a certain disease has caused your symptoms. During a biopsy, the doctor uses a needle to take a small sample of tissue from your liver while you're under a local anaesthetic. Scientists then examine the liver sample under the microscope or subject the biopsy to various laboratory tests. In some cases, doctors perform the biopsy during an ultrasound or CT scan, which guides the needle to the abnormal area.

Although biopsies are the most accurate way to diagnose some liver diseases, they carry risks. For example, the liver has a very rich blood supply. So, a biopsy can cause bleeding. The biopsy needle could also lead to bile leaking. And if you have liver cancer, Cancer Research UK warns, there is a small risk that the malignancy could spread along the 'tunnel' left by the needle. So, you should discuss the risks and benefits with your doctor.

Laparoscopy

During laparoscopy, the surgeon puts a thin tube with a camera and light at the end into your abdomen through a small cut and looks at your liver on a video screen. The surgeon may need to insert the camera at several places around the abdomen to examine your liver from different angles. You'll be under a general anaesthetic and will probably need to stay in hospital overnight.

Liver function tests

As mentioned in Chapter 1, the liver produces numerous enzymes that protect us from the potential hazards that we encounter during our everyday life. Levels of some of these enzymes rise and fall depending on, for example, what chemicals we encounter, whether you drink alcohol excessively, eat a poisonous plant or take some medicines. The liver cannot tell if the chemical is a life-saving medicine or a potentially deadly poison.

Liver damage or inflammation can lead to certain enzymes leaking into your bloodstream. So, levels of these enzymes in the blood will be much higher than normal. That's why doctors perform liver function tests (LFTs) to help diagnose and track your hepatic condition. Depending on your particular circumstances, doctors may look at levels of one or more of several enzymes and other proteins in your blood, including:

- Bilirubin and other waste products that may build up in your blood if your liver is not working properly (see page 17).
- Gamma-glutamyltransferase (GGT), which aids digestion. Increased levels of this enzyme are an early sign of liver disease. Indeed, between 30 and 50 per cent of people who drink alcohol excessively show increased levels of GGT. However, several non-hepatic diseases, such as inflammation of the pancreas (pancreatitis) and conditions affecting the prostate gland, can also trigger a rise in GGT.
- Aspartate aminotransferase (AST) and alanine aminotransferase (ALT), which help process amino acids, the building blocks of protein.
- Alkaline phosphatase (ALP), which is found in particularly high levels in the liver, bile duct, kidneys and bone. So, blocked bile ducts can lead to ALP levels rising.

Abnormal levels of these enzymes do not necessarily indicate liver damage. For example, cells throughout the body produce ALP. And while the liver produces most of the ALT in your blood, several tissues produce AST, including the liver, heart, kidney and brain. In other words, diseases elsewhere in your body can lead to abnormal LFTs – but may still indicate that something is seriously wrong. So, you should take the results seriously.

For example, a study from the UK[3] examined LFTs performed on 13,276 people aged at least 75 years. Of these, around 16 per cent showed at least one abnormal LFT. As Table 3.1 shows, people with even one abnormal LFT were much more likely to die than those with normal levels. Furthermore:

- People with abnormal AST levels were seven times more likely to die from liver disease than those with normal LFTs.
- People with abnormal levels of ALP were six times more likely to die from liver disease.
- People with two or more abnormal LFTs were twice as likely to die from cancer and 17 times more likely to die from liver disease than those with normal tests.

Table 3.1 Proportion of elderly people with abnormal liver function tests and the associated increased risk of mortality[3]

Test	Proportion with an abnormal liver function test (per cent)	Increased risk of death in those with an abnormal liver function test (per cent)
Aspartate aminotransferase (AST)	3	27
Alkaline phosphatase (ALP)	9	47
Bilirubin	5	15

Indeed, abnormal LFTs seem to predict an increased risk of death from a wide range of causes. For instance, the study linked abnormal ALP levels to a greater likelihood of dying from cardiovascular (heart and blood vessels) disease (34 per cent increased risk), cancer (61 per cent) and respiratory (lung) conditions (58 per cent).[3]

However, LFTs are not infallible. For example, up to 70 per cent of people with non-alcoholic liver disease (Chapter 6) have normal LFTs.[1] For a while, I worked in a clinical trial unit that tested new medicines on healthy young men. Doctors checked LFTs to help ensure the volunteers' safety. But we warned volunteers not to eat a curry for a few days before: the spices sometimes sent levels of certain enzymes shooting up. Nevertheless, your doctor should always check whether an abnormal LFT is a 'one-off' or indicates a more serious underlying problem. Don't ignore an abnormal LFT.

Classifying liver disease

As we've seen, doctors choose the most appropriate test from among a range of alternatives to see how well your liver is working. Each test views the liver from a different 'angle', so doctors often combine several tests to grade the damage. The Child–Pugh (sometimes called the Child–Turcotte–Pugh) cirrhosis classification is one of the most widely used 'composite' scores.

Using the Child–Pugh cirrhosis classification, doctors score five key symptoms of liver disease on a three-point scale:

• total levels of bilirubin (page 17);

- level of albumin in the blood (page 9);
- prothrombin time, which measures how quickly your blood clots;
- ascites (page 18);
- hepatic encephalopathy, which, as we have seen, refers to mental changes caused by liver disease.

A person with cirrhosis who has not yet developed ascites has a score of 1. Difficult-to-control ascites score 3. The doctor adds up the total score: the maximum is 15. This allows doctors to gain an insight into your prognosis (Table 3.2). As the table shows, people with cirrhosis are at increased risk of complications after elective or emergency surgery. So, you need to discuss the risks and benefits of any procedure with your doctor.

Table 3.2 Prognosis for patients with liver disease according to the Child–Pugh classification[4]

Class	Points	Life expectancy (years)	Proportion who die after abdominal surgery (per cent)
A	5–6	15–20	10
B	7–9	4–14	30
C	10–15	1–3	80

4

The A to E of viral hepatitis

Reports of jaundice that spread between people date back to ancient Greece. In the eighth century AD, letters between Pope Zacharias and St Boniface mention contagious jaundice. And in the late nineteenth century, around 1 in every 7 German shipyard workers who were treated with a smallpox vaccine manufactured from blood developed jaundice and hepatitis. Doctors soon realized that poorly sterilized syringes and needles could transmit jaundice, a condition that they called serum hepatitis. By 1937, scientists realized that a blood-borne virus (hepatitis B virus) caused serum hepatitis.[1]

Today, we know that five viruses – hepatitis A to E – are among the most common causes of liver disease. All five viruses replicate inside hepatocytes, which damages the cells. Furthermore, as the body tries to eradicate the virus, the immune system targets the infected liver cells. In some cases, this dual attack causes swelling, inflammation (hepatitis), scarring and can be the first step on a road that leads to liver cancer. Indeed, viral hepatitis causes around one-third of new cases of hepatocellular carcinoma, the most common liver cancer, in the UK each year.[2] This chapter introduces the hepatitis viruses and looks at the best way to avoid and live with the infections.

Hepatitis A

Most infections with hepatitis A virus (HAV), discovered in 1973,[3] follow the contamination of food and drink with faeces from an infected person. So, not surprisingly, HAV spreads rapidly when personal hygiene and sanitation are poor: HAV is especially common in the Indian subcontinent, Africa, Central and South America, the Far East and eastern Europe. While the World Health Organization (WHO) estimates that 1.4 million people contract HAV annually, the virus is relatively rare in the UK. According to the Health Protection Agency (HPA), doctors diagnosed 337 cases of HAV in England and Wales during 2009, down from 1,837 in 1997.

HAV does not cause persistent (chronic) liver disease and only rarely kills. Nevertheless, HAV can cause a wide spectrum of unpleasant symptoms, including fever, malaise, poor appetite, diarrhoea, nausea, abdominal discomfort and jaundice. The pattern of symptoms depends on your age. In parts of the world where HAV is common, most people catch the infection in early childhood. Children less than 6 years of age do not usually experience marked HAV symptoms: only 10 per cent develop jaundice, for example, the WHO notes. Symptoms are more common and more severe in adults: more than 70 per cent of older children and adults infected with HAV develop jaundice. Nevertheless, HAV's symptoms usually subside within a few weeks without producing long-term complications. Occasionally, however, full recovery takes several months.

Treating and preventing HAV

There is no specific treatment for HAV – in contrast to HCV, for example. So, prevention is key. If you have HAV don't share towels, and wash your hands thoroughly after going to the toilet and before preparing food. Indeed, it might be worth asking someone else to prepare your family's food. HAV can spread through direct contact with infected blood, although this is a much less common route of transmission than poor hygiene. Nevertheless, it's a good idea not to share eating utensils, toothbrushes, razors and the equipment ('works') used to inject street drugs such as heroin, cocaine and amphetamines. But you cannot contract HAV by casual contact.

Seek help if you inject drugs

If you mainline drugs speak to your GP, contact your local drug treatment services <www.talktofrank.com/need-support> or call the Frank drugs helpline on 0800 776600. If you know someone who injects or abuses drugs in other ways, you should advise them, gently and sympathetically, to seek help. With support, many people can overcome addiction to drugs of abuse, whether they are hooked on nicotine, alcohol or heroin.

Make sure you're careful about sanitation when travelling to countries where HAV is common. It is sensible to:

• boil all drinking water (including water used for brushing teeth) or use bottled water, whether you're staying in luxury hotels or backpacking in hostels;

- avoid ice;
- avoid poorly cooked shellfish, uncooked vegetables, salads and unpeeled fruit;
- drink only pasteurized or sterilized milk;
- wash your hands well and regularly, especially after going to the toilet or preparing food or eating (do not share towels);
- use only your own eating utensils, toothbrushes, razors or any other items that could have blood on them.

Your doctor can vaccinate you against HAV, either alone or with a jab that includes either hepatitis B or typhoid fever. It's worth getting a dual jab if one of the other diseases is common in the part of the world you plan to visit. So, talk to your doctor at least 6 weeks before you plan to travel. You should also discuss HAV vaccination with your doctor if you're at high risk of contracting the virus for other reasons, such as if you:

- are a man who has sex with other men;
- inject heroin or other street drugs;
- work with or near sewage;
- work where hygiene is poor (e.g. homeless shelters);
- have a chronic liver disease;
- have haemophilia.

Haemophilia and hepatitis viruses

Patients with haemophilia may receive medicines made from donated blood to replace the protein they lack (such as factor VIII or factor IX) that normally ensures blood clots properly. Screening donated blood dramatically reduces the risk of contracting HAV and other viruses, but a very small risk remains. Speak to your GP if you think that you should be vaccinated or are unsure.

Hepatitis B

In the 1960s, the American scientist Baruch Blumberg was trying to discover why people in different parts of the world varied in their vulnerability to particular diseases. So, Blumberg's team screened thousands of blood samples for antigens – proteins that trigger immune responses.

As Siddhartha Mukherjee notes in *The Emperor of All Maladies*, one particular antigen caught Blumberg's attention. Initially, the team isolated the so-called Australia (Au) antigen from an Australian Aborigine. Further research showed that the antigen was also common in people from Africa and Asia. By contrast, few people from America or Europe had the Au antigen. Then, in 1966, an Au-negative patient in a clinic in New Jersey suddenly started expressing Au antigen and developed rapidly progressing (fulminant) hepatitis. Further research revealed that the Au antigen was part of a virus that caused liver disease. Researchers discovered the microorganism responsible – hepatitis B virus (HBV) – in 1970[3] and started testing a vaccine in 1979.

Transmission of HBV

Infected blood or body fluids transmit HBV. So you can catch HBV:

- during sex with an infected partner;
- by sharing contaminated equipment to inject street drugs;
- during pregnancy, when an infected mother passes HBV to her unborn child;
- after receiving infected blood transfusions or medical treatments (such as factors to help clotting) made from blood;
- by being accidently stabbed with a needle contaminated with infected blood (people working in hospitals or helping drug addicts or the homeless, and so on, are at particularly high risk of 'needlestick' injuries);
- being tattooed, receiving acupuncture or having body piercing with equipment that has not been sterilized properly.

Shared routes of transmission

Several viruses share HBV's routes of transmission, including HCV (see 'Hepatitis C' in this chapter) and HIV, responsible for AIDS. Indeed, around 80 per cent of HIV-positive people are or have been infected with HBV.[2] So taking steps to avoid one virus helps protect you from others.

HBV is much more common in other parts of the world than in the UK. The WHO estimates that 350 million people are chronically infected with HBV. The virus is especially common in South-East Asia, Africa, the Middle and Far East, as well as southern and eastern Europe. Currently, around 180,000 people in the UK are infected with HBV, a number that grows by around 7,000 annually, largely from immigration of infected people.[2]

The course of HBV

Often the initial HBV infection does not cause symptoms. However, some people develop acute hepatitis between 40 and 160 days after HBV infection. Others experience a flu-like illness, including sore throat, tiredness, joint pains and a loss of appetite. HBV may also cause nausea and vomiting as well as severe abdominal discomfort and jaundice. However, fewer than 1 in 100 infected people die during the initial infection, and symptoms resolve as the immune system clears the virus.

In around 1 in 20 adults and about 9 in 10 children, HBV continues to replicate in liver cells after any initial symptoms resolve. If the immune system does not clear the virus within 6 months of the initial infection, doctors regard the person as having chronic HBV. As many people do not experience symptoms, they are unaware that they have chronic HBV. Nevertheless, they remain infectious and at risk of developing cirrhosis and liver cancer. For example:

- Between 2 and 10 per cent of people infected with HBV develop cirrhosis each year.[2]
- Over 5 years, up to one-fifth (14–20 per cent) of people with chronic HBV and compensated cirrhosis die. Approximately 1 in 20 (6 per cent) HBV-positive people with compensated cirrhosis (page 13) progress to decompensated cirrhosis each year. Over 5 years, about three-quarters (70–80 per cent) of people with decompensated cirrhosis due to HBV die.[2]
- People with chronic HBV are up to 100 times more likely to develop hepatocellular carcinoma (Chapter 7) than the general population.[1] Certain factors further increase the risk of liver cancer following HBV infection, including consuming aflatoxin (page 61) and being simultaneously infected with HCV or some parasites.[1]

Treating and preventing HBV

A growing number of medicines seem to reduce the risk of HBV-related complications, notably interferons and antivirals.

Interferons

The body naturally produces proteins called interferons to help eradicate viral infections. Certain natural interferons directly attack HBV as well as bolstering the immune system's ability to tackle infected hepatocytes.[4] Some people with chronic HBV seem to produce relatively low amounts of natural interferon alfa,[2] which may help explain why the infection persists only in certain people.

Studies elucidating the role of natural interferons inspired drug companies to develop therapeutic versions (such as interferon alfa-2a and interferon alfa-2b) for several diseases including HBV, HCV and certain cancers. However, interferon is a protein. If you swallowed interferon, you would digest it in the same way you break down the steak you had for dinner. As a result, you inject interferon into the layer of fat that lies just under the skin (subcutaneous injection). You'll need to inject interferons for several months to have the best chance of eradicating HBV. More recently, scientists have developed a 'pegylated' version (peginterferon), with a prolonged biological effect that reduces the number of injections required.[2]

Although treatment often lasts many months, it's worth sticking with interferon. For example, in one study, 41 per cent of patients showed normal ALT levels (page 25) after 6 months' treatment with pegylated interferon. Meanwhile, viral load declined in 32 per cent. As mentioned in Chapter 3, doctors regularly measure your viral load to see how well you are responding to treatment.

Interferons are not always suitable. For example, people with advanced liver disease may not be able to receive them. And while serious side effects are uncommon, interferons can cause adverse events including influenza-like symptoms, depression and fatigue.[2]

Antivirals

Some drugs, including adefovir dipivoxil and lamivudine, directly attack HBV. As they are not proteins, antivirals do not need to be injected. They also produce fewer side effects than interferon and are suitable for people with advanced liver disease.

However, antivirals do not work in everyone: between one-fifth and one-half of people infected with HBV respond to adefovir dipivoxil. Furthermore, HBV can mutate, so the antiviral does not work as effectively (resistance). For example, up to one-third of people develop resistance to lamivudine after 1 year's treatment, rising to almost three-quarters (70 per cent) after 5 years. Doctors may suggest adefovir dipivoxil if you develop resistance to lamivudine.[2]

Your doctor will help you decide if lamivudine or adefovir dipivoxil are suitable for you. Antivirals may be appropriate if, for example:

- Other diseases mean you cannot take interferon alfa safely.
- You do not respond adequately to interferon alfa. Doctors will measure your viral load (page 33) to see how well treatment is working.
- Interferon alfa causes intolerable side effects.

As they work through different mechanisms, a combination of antivirals and interferon may give you the best chance of eradicating HBV.[2] You should discuss your treatment options with your doctor.

Vaccination

As ever, prevention is better than cure. Indeed, the HBV vaccine was the first immunization that prevented a specific human cancer.[1] Currently, the NHS suggests vaccinating people at increased risk of catching HBV or who are likely to suffer serious complications if they contract the virus, such as:

- people who inject heroin and other street drugs;
- heterosexual people who change sexual partners frequently;
- men who have sex with men;
- babies born to HBV-positive mothers;
- close family and friends of infected people, including families adopting children from countries where HBV is common;
- patients who need blood transfusions or regularly use medicines made from blood, such as those with haemophilia;
- people with other liver diseases;
- people with chronic kidney disease;
- people travelling to countries where HBV is widespread;
- prisoners and people working in high-risk occupations, including

sex workers, nurses, prison wardens, doctors, dentists and laboratory staff.

If you think you should have the HBV jab, or you are unsure, speak
to your GP or local sexual health and genitourinary medicine clinic
(see NHS Choices for your local service: <www.nhs.uk>). You'll need
three jabs over 4–6 months. Doctors will measure levels of antibody
(page 21) against HBV in your blood 1 month after the third dose
to check that the vaccination has worked. Immunity usually lasts 5
years, after which you'll need a booster jab.

Hepatitis C

Highly sensitive blood tests allow scientists to detect almost everyone infected with HBV. So, by the early 1970s scientists realized
that most people who developed hepatitis after a blood transfusion
were not infected with HBV. They had caught another virus – now
called HCV.[1] Unfortunately, scientists have not yet devised a vaccine
for HCV.

Transmission of HCV

According to the WHO, 170 million people carry HCV. Indeed,
HCV is second only to HBV in causing chronic hepatitis, liver cirrhosis and hepatic cancer worldwide.[1] So, it's worth being especially
careful not to catch HCV when you're visiting high-risk areas. And
such places are not necessarily exotic locales far from the tourist
trail. HCV is more common in Egypt than almost anywhere else in
the world – around 15 per cent of the population is infected.[5]

HCV spreads when blood from an infected person gets into
another person's bloodstream. Indeed, around 93 per cent of people
with HCV in England and Wales contracted the virus through intravenous drug use. People are at especially high risk soon after they
begin injecting drugs, when they are more likely to share 'works'
and are less likely to understand the importance of taking steps
to minimize the risk. Furthermore, many, even most, people who
experiment with injectable drugs do not become addicted long
term. So, doctors do not realize that the person has had a drug
dependency problem and the user is probably unaware that they
have caught HCV.[6]

Blood transfusions and products, sex and other members of the same household can also transmit HCV. But these are rare:

- Blood transfusions are responsible for about 1 in 60 cases.[6] The NHS started screening blood donations for HCV in 1991. Nevertheless, people still acquire HCV from blood transfusions in countries that do not screen donations.
- Around 1 in 70 cases of HCV follow sexual exposure.[6] So, it's worth using condoms, which protect against all sexually transmitted infections.
- Although HCV occasionally spreads among people in the same household, the HPA notes that you can't catch HCV through 'normal social contact'.

The progression of HCV

Soon after infection with HCV you may experience fatigue (which varies from mild to severe) poor appetite, weight loss, depression, anxiety, problems with memory and concentration, pain or discomfort in the abdomen and so on. However, many people do not experience symptoms when they catch HCV.[1]

According to the HPA, approximately 15 to 20 per cent of people clear HCV naturally within 6 months of contracting the virus. In the remainder, the virus can persist for decades. The course of HCV varies widely:

- Many people never develop signs or symptoms and may spend the rest of their life unaware that they carry HCV.
- At least one-quarter of people with chronic HCV develop cirrhosis within 30–40 years of infection.[7]
- Between 1 in 100 and 1 in 25 people with cirrhosis due to HCV develop liver cancer each year. Almost everyone with HCV who develops liver cancer has cirrhosis.[1]

Doctors cannot yet tell who will develop HCV's serious complications. However, HCV generally progresses more rapidly in people who acquire the infection when older and in men. These are not hard-and-fast rules. However, everyone with HCV should limit – and ideally avoid – alcohol. Even moderate alcohol consumption can hasten cirrhosis. Indeed, the combination of HCV and alcohol may exacerbate the damage and hasten the decline in liver function more than you would expect if you simply added the risk factors together. On the other hand, abstinence may reverse some alcohol-related damage, improve the response to treatment and reduce the risk of cirrhosis.[7]

Alcohol and HCV

Up to 70 per cent of people infected with HCV either abuse alcohol or previously had a drinking problem, while around 30 per cent of people with alcoholic liver disease are infected with the virus. Continuing to drink seems to speed the progression to cirrhosis among people infected with HCV. Furthermore, viral load is generally higher in regular than infrequent alcohol drinkers, while alcohol undermines the response to interferon.[8]

Preventing and treating HCV

As there is no vaccine, preventing HCV focuses on good hygiene, such as using disposable sterile needles for body piercing and not sharing toothbrushes, razors and other items that could be contaminated with blood. The HPA also suggests covering wounds and cuts with waterproof dressings and using undiluted bleach to clean up blood spills.[7]

In addition, medicines can eradicate chronic HCV infections in some people. For example, combining interferon (see above) and an antiviral called ribavirin clears HCV in up to 50 per cent of people with the most common form of the virus (genotype 1 – see below) in Europe and North America.[9,10] However, interferons can cause depression and other psychiatric problems, influenza-like symptoms and low levels of some blood cells (cytopenia).[9]

Viral load declines dramatically in the first 24–48 hours after starting interferon alfa. During this time, interferon stops replication of the virus. The rate of decline then slows as the body gradually removes infected liver cells.[11] As a result, treatment lasts many weeks – often almost a year. Doctors regard people with undetectable HCV levels in their blood 24 weeks after the end of treatment as showing a sustained virological response (SVR), raising the prospect (although not, at this point, a guarantee) of a cure.

HCV genotypes

HCV has evolved into six main subtypes, called genotypes. Each genotype encompasses multiple further subtypes (called quasi-species) but these do not need to concern us here. Your genotype can guide treatment:

• Genotype 1 HCV is more difficult to treat than genotype 2 or 3. For example, in people with genotype 1, 48 weeks' treatment with pegylated interferon alfa and ribavirin produces a SVR in 40–50 per cent of cases.[10] However, new antivirals (telaprevir and boceprevir – see below) added to interferon alfa and ribavirin cure around 75 per cent of patients with genotype 1.[9]

• In people with genotype 2 or 3, 24 weeks' treatment with pegylated interferon alfa and ribavirin produces a SVR in 70–80 per cent of cases.[11]

So, your doctor will take a blood sample to determine which genotype you're infected with, the most effective treatment and your probable prognosis.

HCV genotypes around the world

The most common HCV genotype varies around the world. In England, between 2002 and 2007, genotypes 1 (responsible for 45 per cent of cases) and 3 (40 per cent) were more important than types 2 (10 per cent) and 4 (5 per cent).[6] However, genotype 4 accounts for 93 per cent of HCV infections in Egypt.[5]

New antivirals

More recently introduced antivirals – telaprevir and boceprevir – increase the likelihood of SVR in some people with chronic HCV infections. In both cases, patients should not have received HCV therapy before, or their previous treatment should have failed to clear the virus. Treatment with these new antivirals usually lasts around 48 weeks.

The National Institute for Health and Clinical Excellence (NICE) suggests combining telaprevir with peginterferon alfa and ribavirin (triple therapy) for genotype 1 chronic HCV in adults with compensated liver disease (page 13). In one large study, 75 per cent of patients taking triple therapy showed a SVR, compared with 44 per cent of those treated with peginterferon alfa plus ribavirin alone. Telaprevir can cause side effects including: anaemia, rash, itch, diarrhoea, nausea and raised temperature.

NICE recommends triple therapy with boceprevir, peginterferon alfa and ribavirin for adults with genotype 1 chronic HCV and compensated liver disease. In one study, triple therapy with boceprevir increased SVR to between 63 and 66 per cent, compared with 38 per cent with peginterferon alfa-2b and ribavirin alone. Boceprevir's side effects include fatigue, anaemia, nausea, headache and changed taste.

Researchers are developing further generations of antivirals for HCV. In some cases, these seem to be effective in genotype 1, even if peginterferon alfa and ribavirin failed to produce a SVR.[9,10] Although you still need to take precautions, the prospects have never seemed brighter for people with HCV.

Protect yourself from super-infection

Super-infection with other hepatitis viruses – such as contracting both HCV and HAV – often increases the risk of death and disability. In one study, for example, 35 per cent of people with HCV who had HAV super-infection died; a rate 350 times higher than that expected in people without chronic HCV infection.[7] So, doctors may check whether you show antibodies for HAV and HBV. If you have antibodies, you've been infected with that hepatitis virus and, therefore, are already immune. If you don't show antibodies, doctors may suggest vaccinating against hepatitis A or B or both.[7] In some cases, such if you're at high risk, doctors may suggest jabs without testing for antibodies.

Hepatitis D

An outer coat surrounds each hepatitis virus. However, hepatitis D virus (HDV) – sometimes referred to as the delta virus or delta agent – needs HBV to make its coat. In other words, for HDV to replicate in your body you also need to be infected with HBV.

Worldwide, around 1 in 20 people infected with HBV also carry HDV: that's at least 15 million people.[12] The British Liver Trust notes that HDV is most common in central Africa and the Middle

East as well as Central and South America. While HDV is becoming less widespread in some of these areas, immigration means that the number of cases is rising in northern and central Europe.[13]

Contracting HDV dramatically worsens your prospects compared to being infected with HBV alone. For example:

- People infected with both HBV and HDV are some 137 times more likely to develop hepatocellular carcinoma (Chapter 7) than those infected with neither virus.
- People with HBV and HDV are about six times more likely to develop hepatocellular carcinoma than those with HBV alone.[12]

But the risk that these serious complications will emerge partly depends on when you caught HDV. You can acquire HDV at the same time as HBV (co-infection). As 95 per cent of adults clear HBV, they also clear HDV.[13] Alternatively, you may catch HDV after HBV (super-infection), which is especially likely to end in severe chronic hepatitis and cirrhosis.

Only a small amount of blood or body fluid is needed to transmit HDV, so it is commonly spread by intravenous drug use, sex and within families. In some cases, interferon may eradicate HDV or normalize liver function tests. However, interferon does not always work.[13] So, as scientists have not developed a vaccine, good hygiene is the best way to avoid HDV.

Hepatitis E

Hepatitis E virus (HEV) usually produces mild symptoms and rarely causes chronic infection. Patients infected with HEV may develop the characteristic symptoms of viral hepatitis, such as jaundice, dark-brown urine, pale clay-coloured stools, tiredness, fever, nausea, vomiting, abdominal pain and appetite loss. Few people experience all these symptoms, which usually develop around 40 days after infection (although this may vary from 2 weeks to 2 months) and resolve within 1–4 weeks. In rare cases, however, HEV can rapidly prove fatal, particularly in pregnant women.

In common with HAV, HEV spreads from the faecal contamination of food and water. The HPA notes that doctors traditionally believed that people almost always contracted HEV in countries where sanitation is often poor, such as Asia, Africa and Central

America. However, in recent years doctors have diagnosed an increasing number of cases in people who have not travelled to high-risk areas. This might, in part, reflect the growing number of laboratories that are testing for the virus. For example, humans may acquire HEV from infected pigs.

As most people clear HEV naturally, doctors do not specifically treat the infection. However, you should avoid alcohol during the illness, the HPA advises. Pregnant and older people, those with weakened immune systems, and people with chronic liver disease might experience more severe symptoms. So, doctors tend to keep a closer eye on vulnerable people.

Once again, prevention is the best way to avoid HEV:

- Boil all drinking water, including water used for brushing teeth, or use bottled water.
- Avoid ice, poorly cooked shellfish, uncooked vegetables, salads, unpeeled fruit or unpasteurized milk.
- During the illness, and especially during the first 2 weeks, do not prepare meals for other people.
- The HPA advises limiting contact with others, especially with pregnant women and people with chronic liver disease.
- Wash your hands thoroughly with soap and warm water and dry properly after contact with an infected person or their soiled articles.
- Wash hands after going to the toilet, before preparing or serving food or before eating meals.

Indeed, good hygiene is one of the best defences against all five hepatitis viruses.

5

Alcoholic liver disease

The sight of the nation's youth sprawled senselessly drunk on the streets of our towns and cities each weekend, the rising tide of liver disease and the burden imposed by alcohol-related injuries on already stretched casualty departments are eloquent testaments to the harm caused by excessive drinking. Indeed, one-quarter of admissions to intensive care units in Scotland in 2009 were alcohol related[1] and alcohol causes around 1 in every 25 cancers in the UK.[2] Yet tackling alcohol abuse engenders considerable political handwringing as politicians try to balance public health against the personal choice to drink a pint of bitter, sip whisky or savour a glass of Chardonnay.

Tragically, however, drinking alcohol is not always a matter of choice. Alcohol dependency erodes the drinker's ability to say no. The compulsion to drink alcohol overwhelms the dependent person's best intentions, laying siege to every intellectual, rational and emotional defence the drinker can muster, until they can no longer resist alcohol's assault.

Indeed, although alcohol is legal, drinking kills far more people than street drugs. Between 1992 and 2008 in the UK, mortality linked directly to alcohol almost doubled in the UK, from 6.9 to 12.8 for every 100,000 people in the population.[1] In 2008, drug misuse killed 1,738 people in England. But there were 8,664 alcohol-related deaths in 2009, more than double the 4,023 recorded during 1992. The current death toll from alcohol is equivalent to a jumbo jet crashing every 17 days.

Against this background, alcohol accounts from more than one-third (37 per cent) of deaths from liver disease, according to a 2012 report from the National End of Life Care Intelligence Network. To look at the death toll another way: liver disease accounts for around 1 in 10 deaths among people in their 40s – and alcohol abuse is responsible for most of the mortality.

But heavy drinkers don't just harm themselves – alcohol abuse can irreconcilably damage families or cause accidents that injure or kill others. If you know someone who is abusing alcohol you should, gently and sympathetically, advise them to seek help. We'll look at some suggestions to cut down the amount of alcohol you drink later in the chapter.

A nation of heavy drinkers

As these sobering statistics suggest, the UK is a nation of heavy drinkers. According to figures published by the Office for National Statistics in 2011, 38 per cent of people in managerial and professional households drank more than the recommended maximum (4 units for men; 3 units for women) on at least one day in the previous week. This compares with 28 per cent in 'routine' or manual-work households. Furthermore, 19 per cent and 15 per cent, respectively, drank harmful amounts of alcohol (8 units for men; 6 units for women) on at least one day in the last week.

A UK unit of alcohol

One UK unit of alcohol contains 8 g alcohol. So:

- Half a pint of normal strength beer, lager or cider equals 1 unit.
- One small (100 ml) glass of wine equals 1 unit.
- A large (175 ml) glass of wine equals 2 units.
- A single (25 ml) measure of spirits equals 1 unit.
- One 275 ml bottle of alcopop (5.5 per cent/volume) equals 1.5 units.

Some studies and websites refer to an American 'drink', which contains 14 g of alcohol or just less than two UK units.

In other words, millions of people regularly put their health at risk by drinking excessively. Indeed, heavy drinking increases your likelihood of developing several serious conditions, including heart attacks, strokes and several malignancies.[3]

But these are not the only health problems caused by heavy drinking. Because the liver metabolizes alcohol, removing about 1 unit from your blood every hour, it is especially vulnerable to alcohol's assault. For example:

- The risk of developing cirrhosis doubles once alcohol consumption exceeds 50 g alcohol daily and increases approximately fivefold among those drinking more than 100 g a day.[4]
- Most people who drink heavily for several years develop fatty livers (Chapter 6). Alcoholic drinks are often packed with calories, and so contribute to obesity.
- Between 10 and 35 per cent of people who drink heavily for several years show alcohol-related hepatitis, and 8 and 20 per cent develop cirrhosis.[5]

Once alcoholic liver damage emerges, continuing to drink dramatically worsens your prospects. For example:

- About 90 per cent of people with compensated cirrhosis (page 13) due to alcohol live for 5 years if they abstain from drinking.
- Survival declines to less than 70 per cent if people with compensated cirrhosis persistently drink.
- Five-year survival declines to, at most, 30 per cent in people who continue to drink after developing alcohol-related decompensated (page 13) liver disease.[5] That's a worse outlook than for many cancers.
- Drinking excessively for a long time undermines the prospects for people with non-alcoholic liver diseases, such as HCV (page 35).

Why alcohol damages your liver

Each person's body responds to alcohol abuse in a different way. In many people, heavy drinking can cause fatty liver, inflammation (alcoholic hepatitis) and cirrhosis. Yet many people never develop signs or symptoms of liver disease, despite years of excessive consumption. On the other hand, some people develop alcoholic liver disease and cirrhosis even if they have never been dependent on drink. Clearly, the amount you drink is not the only risk factor.[5]

Indeed, scientists still do not fully understand the complex mechanisms by which alcohol damages the liver (see box 'Changes linked to alcoholic liver disease'). However, at least part of your risk – probably around 50 to 60 per cent – of developing alcoholic liver disease or becoming addicted to drink depends on the genes you inherited from your biological parents. For example, people who are genetically predisposed to produce enzymes that break down alcohol more effectively are less likely to suffer liver damage or become addicted than those with less effective metabolisms. Other people may be genetically 'programmed' to repair the damage caused by excessive alcohol consumption more efficiently or better able to mop up tissue-damaging free radicals (see page 56) generated by chronic alcohol consumption.[5]

Changes linked to alcoholic liver disease

Researchers have identified numerous changes that seem to increase the risk of liver damage, as these selected examples show.[5]

- Alcohol markedly reduces hepatocytes' ability to generate the energy that liver cells need to fuel their activity. So, liver cells are more likely to die or be too inactive to meet the body's demands.
- Many systems that the body uses to break down alcohol create a chemical called acetaldehyde, which poisons liver and other cells.
- Alcohol increases levels of free radicals (page 56) while simultaneously undermining the body's defences against these tissue-damaging chemicals.
- Alcohol increases the amount of fat in the liver (Chapter 6).
- Alcohol impairs immune defences.

Further studies are needed to characterize the contribution made by each of these changes to alcoholic liver disease.

Diet and alcoholic liver disease

Often, people who abuse alcohol don't eat healthily, which makes liver damage even more likely. For instance, people who abuse alcohol may replace calories from nutritious food with 'empty' calories from ethanol (the alcohol in alcoholic drinks). And many people who drink excessively may not eat sufficient antioxidants, such as vitamins A, C and E.[5] So, free radicals are more likely to ravage the cells in their liver and elsewhere in their body. Indeed, before the 1970s, many doctors believed that poor diets, rather than excessive drinking, caused alcoholic cirrhosis.

Patients with alcoholic liver disease are often also deficient in other vitamins, including folic acid (vitamin B_9), which the body converts into folate; thiamine (vitamin B_1); and pyridoxine (vitamin B$_6$). These deficiencies can increase the risk of anaemia, poor mental agility and night blindness.[5]

The dangers of drinking during pregnancy

Drinking excessively during pregnancy can cause fetal alcohol syndrome (FAS), which is characterized by hallmark facial features such as a smooth cleft from the nose to upper lip, abnormalities in the opening for the eye between the upper and lower eyelids, and a thin upper lip. Affected children also typically show impaired growth and mental problems. The National Organisation for Foetal Alcohol Syndrome (NOFAS-UK) suggests that 6,000–7,000 children are born in Britain each year with FAS and related milder versions of the condition – that's roughly 1 per cent of babies. The NHS suggests that pregnant women and those trying to conceive should avoid alcohol. At most, you should drink 1 or 2 units once or twice a week.

Am I drinking excessively?

Clearly, you need to keep your alcohol consumption within safe limits. And women cannot safely drink as much alcohol as men – especially if you are pregnant or trying for children. The NHS recommends not regularly drinking more than 3–4 units a day if you're a man or 2–3 units daily if you're a women (regularly means every or most days). Indeed, almost all men who usually drink more than 40–80 g of alcohol a day (5–10 units) for between 10 and 12 years develop alcoholic liver disease. In women, consuming more than 20–40 g a day (2.5–5 units) for 10–12 years makes alcoholic liver disease almost inevitable.[5]

Scientists still do not fully understand why women develop cirrhosis and other alcohol-related liver damage at around half the level of consumption as men. However, studies have offered some clues. For example, female hormones (such as oestrogen) may reduce the ability of some enzymes to break down alcohol. Furthermore, blood levels of ethanol are higher in women than men if they drink the same amount, partly because women tend to be lighter and have more body fat.[5] Fat, unlike muscle, does not absorb much alcohol. So, more alcohol remains in the blood.

So, how can you tell if you are abusing alcohol? The CAGE questionnaire is one of the most widely used tests for excessive drinking.

If you answer yes to two or more of these questions you may have an alcohol problem:

C: Have you ever felt you should **cut down** on your drinking?
A: Have people ever **annoyed** you by criticizing your drinking?
G: Have you ever felt bad or **guilty** about your drinking?
E: **Eye opener**: Have you ever had a drink first thing in the morning to steady your nerves or to get rid of a hangover?

However, CAGE is not perfect. The 'ever' phrase means that the questionnaire captures people who had a drink problem, but now abstain or keep their drinking within recommended levels. Furthermore, most people tend to deny that they abuse alcohol until health, social or legal problems emerge. In other words, CAGE and most other tests tend to detect problems associated with drinking rather than whether the person is drinking excessively. So it's also worth keeping a note of the amount you drink.

Cutting down your drinking

Most people want to try to tackle their drink problem themselves before going to see a doctor or joining a support group. So how can you make a start?

The first step is to keep a diary over a month or so in which you note how much you drink and when (places and circumstances, such as when you're feeling down or stressed out). According to a 2009 report by Alcohol Concern, the average adult drinker under-estimates their consumption by the equivalent of a bottle of wine each week (a 750 ml bottle of 12 per cent wine contains 9 units). So don't guess and be honest.

You may find that keeping a note means that you start cutting down. If you get so drunk that you can't recall how much you drank the night before, you almost certainly have a problem. Returning to your old pattern after abstaining for a while is another common characteristic of alcohol abuse.

Indeed, your drinking pattern offers another clue. Most people vary their drinking pattern. People who abuse alcohol tend to drink more regularly, partly because they need to stave off withdrawal symptoms, which often peak between 24 and 48 hours after the last drink, and can include tremor (the shakes), insomnia, agitation, depression and even fits.

Drinking safely

If you already have liver disease or any other serious condition, it's a good idea to talk your plans over with your doctor. You (and if appropriate your doctor) should set a goal. Some people who drink heavily will need to abstain, probably for the rest of their life, especially if they have liver disease. However, other people find that they can cut back and drink within the recommended limit – but they need to remain alert for changes in their drinking habits. Obviously, if you have liver disease or any other health problem, you should follow your doctor's advice about your safe drinking limits. Your personalized limit may differ from the government's recommendation.

You also need to think about why you drink and be honest about the benefits it brings or brought you. Some people abuse alcohol because they are depressed, anxious (page 117) or have another psychiatric condition. While drowning sorrows in alcohol brings a short-lived relief from the mental torment, alcohol often makes matters much worse. If you're depressed over your finances or a dysfunctional marriage, for example, alcohol can fuel the problem: alcohol's not cheap and drunken behaviour can undermine relationships. And the lack of inhibitions may mean you say or do things that you'll bitterly regret for the rest of your life. Alcohol's a depressant, so the hangover often exacerbates your melancholia. Your GP can help you tackle any underlying mental torment with drugs, counselling or both.

Jack's story

Jack worked for 15 years as a successful and well-liked sales representative for an engineering company. Following a hostile takeover, the directors announced a widespread 'rationalization'. However, at the time, Jack was recovering from the breakdown of his 10-year marriage 6 months previously – and his sales figures had slipped. Jack felt depressed, anxious and worried and found it harder and harder to evoke the jovial, optimistic frame of mind he needed to sell. So, he started drinking heavily in the pub after work and in hotel bars during sales trips.

As his drinking worsened, he felt his judgement slip and he missed some big contracts. And, once a legend in the company for his punctuality, he began missing appointments and taking more time off sick to nurse his hangovers. After losing his job, Jack decided to ask his doctor for help tackling his depression and drinking. Blood tests showed his liver enzymes were dangerously elevated. However, there were no signs of cirrhosis. A now teetotal Jack is now making a success of a new job and a new relationship.

How you then progress is up to you. Some people pick a day and decide that they will stop or dramatically cut down. Other people find that it's easier to gradually reduce the amount they drink. (It's especially important to keep a diary if you're slowly cutting down – to make sure you don't slip back into bad ways.) However, even if you plan to return to drinking safe levels of alcohol, it's worth 'drying out' and not drinking for at least a month to allow your liver a chance to recover. If you can't stop drinking for a few weeks, you might have an alcohol problem. Taking milk thistle (page 105) may help your liver recover.

Tricks to reduce consumption

Various tricks can help you slowly reduce your alcohol consumption:

- Check the number of units in a drink before you buy it; favour drinks with a lower alcohol content. For example, avoid wine with alcohol by volume (ABV) of 14 or 15 per cent. Try to buy bottles containing around 10 per cent ABV.
- Replace large wine glasses with smaller ones.
- If you prefer spirits, buy a measure so you can tell how many units of gin you're adding to your tonic or fingers of whisky you're pouring at home.
- Only drink alcohol with a meal.
- Alternate alcoholic beverages with either water or soft drinks. This slows your alcohol consumption and helps avoid dehydration.
- Mix your drink – try spritzers and shandies rather than wine and beer, and water down or increase the amount of mixers you add to spirits.
- Quench your thirst with a soft drink rather than an alcoholic beverage.
- Make sure you have dry (drink-free) days each week. As we'll see,

the power of 'cues' means that you may need to avoid your usual haunts and drinking partners on your dry days.
- Find a hobby that does not involve drinking.

Deciding whether or not to tell your family, friends and colleagues that you're trying to cut down on alcohol can be difficult. Some family and friends offer you advice and support, especially if they have previously expressed concerns about your drinking. But they may not be as understanding if you slip back: it's easy to underestimate how addictive alcohol can sometimes prove. However, some people may feel that you are challenging their drinking habits, and may prove hostile or condescending, especially if some of your social or work life revolves around drinking.

Nevertheless, you can cut down, without antagonizing friends and colleagues. For example:

- Offer to be the designated driver or say you have an early start in the morning. (It's worth noting that you may still be over the drink–drive limit in the morning after an especially heavy session.)
- Tell a white lie and claim that you're on medication and your doctor has advised you not to drink. If asked why, just say: 'I'd rather not talk about it at the moment, it's the wrong time and place.'
- When you're out with a large group, buying drinks in rounds can rapidly rack up the amount you consume. The group tends to keep pace with the fastest drinker. Try to buy rounds only when you're in small groups.
- Have soft drinks between the alcoholic drinks. You can ask for bottles of beer, shandies and spritzers, or halves instead of pints. You could offer to buy the round when your glass is half full and ask the bar staff to top up your glass with a half pint.
- Eat before you start drinking and regularly have snacks. Food slows the speed at which you absorb alcohol.

In addition, several books and websites (see 'Useful addresses') can help you reduce your drinking. If you feel you really can't quit without help, your doctor can refer you to alcohol services on the NHS. Doctors may also, for example, offer drugs to help you deal with cravings as well as 'talking therapies' and counselling that help you understand why you drink, how to cut down and the best way to deal with difficult situations. Alcoholics Anonymous and other support groups help many people, although they are not for everyone. But there is plenty of help available. The most difficult step is accepting that you need help – and asking for assistance.

Understanding why you drink

If you find cutting down tough, you should ask yourself some searching questions. You could keep a journal (such as a password-protected computer file) to record your thoughts. I would suggest you keep it to yourself – the insights are deeply personal and may mean considering your attitudes towards, and relationships with, other people. However, such insights can be invaluable: after all, people start drinking because alcohol (indeed, using any drug whether legal or illicit) brings benefits, even if it is helping in social situations, to unwind or to offer a brief respite from mental torment.

So, it's worth asking yourself why you drink and trying to find an alternative. If stress triggers your drinking, try to bolster your defences with meditation, exercise and so on. If you're depressed (page 117) speak to your doctor. If you endure financial or relationship problems, consider seeking help from debt or marriage counsellors.

Keeping a diary will also help you identify your triggers. You'll be vulnerable to situations that addiction experts call cues: in other words, circumstances, places and emotions that you associate with drinking and that stimulate the desire for alcohol. So, walking past your local can trigger an urge for a pint, a meal in a favourite restaurant can trigger a desire for a bottle of wine or a stressful meeting can trigger the desire for a slug of whisky. (Try to find a way home that avoids the opportunity to drink after a tough day.) Obviously, it's a good idea to avoid these cues as far as possible.

Alcohol is such a part of most people's everyday life that it's easy to underestimate the harm that excessive drinking causes, the numbers of lives it damages and the pain it causes. If you have liver disease, you may need to become teetotal. If not, you need to ensure you keep your consumption in check – for the sake of your liver and your health and well-being generally.

6

Non-alcoholic liver disease

Walk down any high street and it's soon clear from the double chins, sagging bottoms and bulging waistbands that too many of us carry too much weight. Indeed, around three-fifths of women and two-thirds of men in the UK are overweight or obese. Many over-weight people find buying fashionable clothes difficult, changing in public embarrassing and even mild exercise tough going. But the problems posed by excess weight are more than skin deep.

Excess weight causes or contributes to numerous serious diseases, including heart disease, type 2 diabetes mellitus (T2DM; the type that usually emerges during middle age) and some malignancies. Indeed, according to the *British Journal of Cancer*, excess body weight caused about 1 in every 18 cancers in the UK during 2010.[1] But the health burden imposed by excess weight is going to get even heavier. If current trends continue, another 11 million adults in the UK will be obese by 2030, resulting in 331,000 extra cases of coronary heart disease and strokes, 545,000 more cases of diabetes and 87,000 additional cancers.

Obesity and liver damage

The liver is not immune to damage caused by the fat of the land. A healthy liver contains very little or no fat. However, as your weight rises, fat begins to deposit in the liver. Over time, the gradual accu-mulation of fat can cause a condition called non-alcoholic fatty liver disease (NAFLD).

Not surprisingly, given our bulging waistbands, NAFLD is the leading cause of chronic liver damage in Western countries. Overall, between one-fifth and one-third of people have NAFLD. However, almost all (95 per cent) obese people and three-quarters of people with diabetes have NAFLD.[2] According to the British Liver Trust, NAFLD usually emerges around the age of 50 years and is more common in men than women.

But NAFLD does not necessarily leave your liver with the consistency of *foie gras*. Doctors generally diagnose NAFLD when your liver contains more than 5 per cent fat – that's just 60–75g for an average liver.[3] They will diagnose NAFLD only after excluding other factors that could cause fatty liver, such as alcohol abuse, viral hepatitis or certain medicines.[4] So, doctors typically diagnose NAFLD only if the patient drinks less than 10 g of alcohol a day (a UK unit contains 8 g of alcohol). If doctors think that alcohol is the main cause or a very important contributor to your hepatic symptoms, they will diagnose alcoholic liver disease (Chapter 5). However, the progression of NAFLD is broadly similar to that of alcoholic liver disease.

In addition to excess weight, several diseases can contribute to fatty liver, the British Liver Trust notes, including:

- dangerously high blood pressure (hypertension);
- having been malnourished, starved or given nutrition intravenously (into a vein);
- having too much cholesterol and triglyceride in the blood (hyperlipidaemia). Indeed, triglycerides (page 8) account for most of the fat in NAFLD.

Furthermore, fat-filled cells can also store certain toxins,[5] which may exacerbate liver damage.

The progression of NAFLD

Initially at least, fatty liver does not cause symptoms. So, you may be unaware that you've taken the first steps on a path that could end in liver failure or cancer. An accumulation of fat in the liver that does not cause symptoms is called steatosis.

In some cases, the fat deposits trigger inflammation in and around the liver cells – so-called non-alcoholic steatohepatitis (NASH). As a result, patients experience swelling of, and discomfort or pain around, the liver. Over time, NASH can scar the liver. As we've seen before, fibrosis (scarring) can progress to cirrhosis, irreversible liver damage and liver cancer:

- One study that followed NASH patients for almost 6 years found that between 26 and 37 per cent developed fibrosis and up to 9 per cent showed cirrhosis.[6]

- Overall, 4–27 per cent of NASH cases transform into hepatocellular carcinoma (page 60).[6]
- NASH raises the risk of liver cancer by up to tenfold.[7]

Diagnosing NAFLD

As the early stages rarely cause symptoms, doctors often detect NAFLD when they feel an enlarged liver or detect mild changes in liver function tests (page 24) during a physical examination.[3] Doctors use a liver biopsy (page 24) to distinguish NASH from simple steatosis. Under the microscope, a liver sample from a person with NASH shows fat, inflammation and damaged liver cells.

NAFLD and diabetes

Excess weight causes about 9 in every 10 cases of T2DM, which, according to Diabetes UK, accounts for between 85 and 90 per cent of the 2.9 million cases of diabetes in the UK. T2DM usually occurs in obese and overweight people who are more than 40 years old. However, in South Asian and black people, T2DM typically appears from the age of 25 years and Diabetes UK estimates that up to 1,400 children in the UK have T2DM. NAFLD tends to be particularly aggressive in people with diabetes.[4] This link seems to be one reason why diabetes increases the risk of hepatocellular carcinoma between 1.86-fold and 4-fold.[6]

Treating NAFLD

The decline from steatosis to cancer is not inevitable. For example, the study that followed patients for almost 6 years found that liver damage improved in between 18 and 29 per cent of people with NASH and remained stable in the remainder.[6] And you can take steps to prevent or slow the decline.

Doctors have yet to find a medicine that treats NAFLD, although several studies are underway. So doctors generally suggest that patients:

- increase exercise, which burns fat (page 96);
- eat a low-fat, healthy diet (Chapter 9);
- avoid alcohol (Chapter 5);

- avoid unnecessary medicines (page 80);
- lose weight (page 94).

Indeed, gradually losing weight by combining diet and exercise can stop or reverse liver damage in NASH patients and improve liver function tests: losing 4.5–6.8 kg (10–15 lb) often returns levels of liver transaminases (page 25) to normal.[3] And, of course, losing weight has numerous other health benefits. However, as with any serious medical condition, if you are a NASH patient you should speak to a doctor before changing your diet or exercise patterns.

Tackling free radicals

High levels of free radicals seem to contribute to the liver damage in NASH. Indeed, on average, people with NASH have low blood levels of vitamin E. NASH patients also tend to have lower levels of certain carotenoids (yellow, orange and red pigments in plants) that reduce the damage from free radicals in their blood, including:

- beta-carotene, the orange pigment in carrots, which the body converts to vitamin A (as we mentioned in Chapter 1, the liver stores vitamin A);
- lutein, a carotenoid in green leafy vegetables such as spinach and kale;
- lycopene, found in tomatoes.[8]

These 'antioxidant' nutrients mop up tissue-damaging free radicals. The growing number of studies linking free radicals to NASH prompted researchers to investigate various antioxidants to prevent the damage caused by fatty liver.

So, it's a good idea to eat foods rich in carotenoids and vitamin E. You could also think about a supplement – after speaking to your doctor first, if you've been diagnosed with chronic liver disease or another serious ailment. One study compared 800 IU vitamin E a day with a placebo (a pill that looks identical but which does not contain any active medicine). After taking the supplement for 96 weeks, twice as many people in the vitamin E group showed an improvement in NASH compared with the placebo group (43 per cent and 19 per cent, respectively). People in the vitamin E group also showed improved blood ALT and AST levels (page 25) as well as reduced amounts of fat and inflammation in the liver.[9]

Free radicals

A slice of apple left exposed to the air soon turns brown. A group of tissue-damaging chemicals called free radicals causes the colour change. In the body, free radicals can damage tissues, cells and even our genetic code (DNA). Unfortunately, free radicals are all around us. Our body forms free radicals as by-products of the normal chemical reactions that keep us alive. Our immune system uses free radicals to destroy invading bacteria. And pollution, cigarette smoke, pesticides and even sunlight can generate free radicals.

Why are free radicals so dangerous? You may know that, put rather simply, electrons orbit the nucleus of an atom, rather like planets orbit a star. Electrons are most stable in pairs. As a result, a molecule or atom with a 'spare' electron – a free radical – will try to restore balance by 'stealing' an electron. This damages the 'donor', such as fat, DNA or protein, and may even kill the cell. That's why free radicals seem to increase the risk of developing several serious conditions, including heart disease, cancer, strokes, Alzheimer's disease and rheumatoid arthritis.

You could boost your intake of foods that are rich in vitamin E, such as:

- nuts and seeds – almonds, hazelnuts and pine nuts are good sources;
- vegetable oils, such as olive, safflower or sunflower oil. Ideally, use cold-pressed vegetable oils: cold pressing removes less vitamin E than some other processing methods;
- green leafy vegetables;
- fortified cereals and spreads (read the label);
- mackerel, salmon – in addition to vitamin E, fish contains high levels of a fat that may help improve NAFLD (page 88).

Tackling diabetes

As we have already seen, many NASH patients have other diseases or risk factors, such as diabetes, high blood pressure or raised cholesterol levels, which your doctor may suggest treating. In addition, some lifestyle advice for treating NASH, such as weight loss, also helps tackle these concurrent conditions. For example, NICE suggests that overweight people with type 2 diabetes should aim to lose between 5 and 10 per cent of their body weight to reduce the risk of complications, such as heart disease, loss of vision and amputations.

Microvascular and macrovascular complications

Doctors broadly separate diabetic complications into microvascular and macrovascular:

- Microvascular complications include neuropathy (nerve damage), nephropathy (kidney disease) and retinopathy (damage to the light-sensitive layer at the back of eye).
- Macrovascular complications include heart disease, stroke and peripheral vascular disease (a blockage in the blood vessels supplying the limbs, which can end in gangrene and amputation of the toes, feet and lower leg).

Other complications include a higher risk of infections, impotence, problems during pregnancy and, in children, impaired growth and development.

NASH shows a particularly close relationship with diabetes and insulin resistance (which emerges before full-blown T2DM.) Cells use a sugar called glucose to fuel their activities. The hormone insulin stimulates cells to take glucose from the blood. The cell then uses the glucose to generate energy. (You can learn more about diabetes and its treatment in *The Diabetes Healing Diet* by Christine Craggs-Hinton and myself). As T2DM progresses, muscle, liver, fat and other cells gradually respond less and less well to insulin, so these insulin-resistant cells take up less glucose from the blood. As a result, glucose levels in the blood rise, which, over time, can cause microvascular and macrovascular complications.

The body tries to reduce blood glucose levels by flushing the excess out of the body. So, people with diabetes urinate more.

Medieval doctors regularly inspected their patients' urine by holding a sample in a bulbous glass flask to the light. Some went further: they took a swig. In 1674, the English physician Thomas Willis used the sweet taste to distinguish diabetes from other causes of frequent urination, such as infections. You don't need to resort to tasting your urine, but you should see your doctor you have any of the symptoms in Table 6.1.

Table 6.1 Common symptoms of diabetes

More frequent urination than usual, especially during the night

Increased thirst; drinking excessively

Extreme tiredness and fatigue

Unexplained weight loss

Genital itching or regular episodes of thrush

Cuts and wounds that heal slowly

Blurred vision

Source: Adapted from Diabetes UK

Insulin resistance and NASH

Against this background, scientists are trying to determine whether reducing insulin resistance improves NASH. For example, metformin, one of the most widely used drugs for T2DM, decreases glucose production by the liver and increases its uptake by cells. Another drug, called pioglitazone (which reduces insulin resistance in the liver), improved NASH, but was less effective than vitamin E: 34 and 43 per cent of patients improved, respectively, compared with 19 per cent taking placebo. Pioglitazone improved levels of ALT and AST in the blood (page 25) as well as reducing the amount of fat and inflammation in the liver.[9]

More research is needed to determine how well insulin sensitizers work in NASH. However, if you have concurrent diabetes these drugs reduce your risk of developing complications. So, you should take antidiabetic medications as prescribed by your doctor. Nevertheless, keeping a healthy weight and following a healthy lifestyle are set to remain the best defences against NASH.

7

Liver cancer

Liver cancer accounts for about 1 in every 100 malignancies in the UK. According to Cancer Research UK, doctors diagnosed 3,594 liver cancers in the UK during 2008. Unfortunately, most people with liver cancer face a bleak future.

In the UK, 3,618 people died from the malignancy during 2009 – roughly the same number as were diagnosed with liver cancer. In parts of the world where advanced treatments are not available, such as rural areas in China and Africa, survival is typically only 4 months once symptoms emerge.[1] Even in the UK, only around one-fifth (20 per cent) of people are alive a year after being diagnosed with liver cancer. Just 1 in 20 people (5 per cent) live for at least 5 years, Cancer Research UK comments. Nevertheless, you can reduce your risk of developing liver cancer. And provided doctors diagnose liver cancer early enough, modern treatments occasionally cure this deadly malignancy.

Cancer: cells out of control

Normally cells divide, under tight control, to replace old and damaged tissue. The old or damaged cells then die. In some cases, however, damaged cells do not die, new cells form when they should not, or both. Accumulations of these extra cells create a swelling, called a tumour.

A tumour is not necessarily cancerous. Some cancers (such as leukaemia, a blood malignancy arising in bone marrow) do not create a tumour. In other cases, the accumulation of cells creates a 'benign' tumour that is not cancerous and, usually, does not recur after a surgeon removes the mass of cells. Importantly, benign tumours do not invade the surrounding tissue or spread to other parts of the body (metastasize). Several benign tumours can grow in the liver:

- Haemangiomas are the most common benign liver tumours

and start in blood vessels. Usually they do not need treatment. However, a surgeon may remove the tumour if it starts bleeding.

- Hepatic adenomas begin in hepatocytes and, in a few people, cause pain, create a lump in the abdomen or bleed. As hepatic adenomas can rupture, causing severe blood loss, and there is a small risk they could transform into a cancer, a doctor may suggest they are removed.
- Focal nodular hyperplasia (FNH) is a mass of several different types of cell, including hepatocytes and bile duct cells. Doctors often can find distinguishing FNH from liver cancers difficult and so may remove the growth as a precaution.

By contrast, cancerous cells divide and grow uncontrollably, and unlike benign tumours, invade the surrounding healthy tissue. In time, most cancers spread in the blood or lymph to other parts of the body, forming secondary tumours called metastases. So, doctors distinguish primary from secondary liver cancers. Most cancers are named after the organ from which they first emerge. So, primary hepatocellular carcinomas first develop in hepatocytes. Secondary liver cancers spread from a primary malignancy elsewhere in the body. For example, primary breast, lung or bowel cancers commonly produce liver metastases. But the doctor will still classify the secondary liver malignancies as, for example, metastatic breast cancer.

Secondary liver cancers are examples of 'visceral' metastases, which can carry a particularly poor prognosis. For example, in a study of 470 women with breast cancer, 73 per cent of those with a single secondary cancer in their skeleton survived for 5 years. This compared with 22 per cent of those with liver, lung and other visceral metastases.[2]

Types of liver cancer

Almost any cell in the body can become cancerous. But some cells are more likely to turn malignant than others. For example, according to Cancer Research UK, about 85 per cent of liver cancers are hepatocellular carcinomas (HCC): in other words, the malignancy arises in hepatocytes (page 3). Indeed, worldwide, HCC is the sixth most common malignancy and the third leading cause of cancer death.[3] Less common liver cancers include:

- cholangiocarcinoma – a cancer that arises in the bile ducts;
- angiosarcoma – a cancer affecting blood vessels in the liver. Angiosarcoma generally occurs in people in their 70s and 80s;
- hepatoblastoma – a very rare cancer affecting young children.

Risk factors for liver cancer

Between 70 and 90 per cent of HCCs develop in people with chronic liver disease.[3] For example:

- Overall, one-third of people with cirrhosis develop HCC.[4] Indeed, HCC is the leading cause of death among people with cirrhosis.[3]
- HBV causes just over half (54 per cent) of HCCs worldwide.
- HCV causes around 31 per cent of HCCs worldwide.
- Each year, between 1 and 3 people in every 500 (0.2–0.6 per cent) who are infected with HBV but have not progressed to cirrhosis develop HCC. The risk rises to 1 in 50 of HBV-infected people who have developed cirrhosis.[3]
- Between 10 and 25 per cent of people with chronic HBV eventually develop HCC.[3]
- Between 3 and 8 per cent of people with HCV who progress to cirrhosis develop HCC annually.[3]

As we saw in Chapter 4, the risk of contracting hepatitis viruses varies across the world. Partly as a result, the importance of the various triggers for HCC differs from country to county. HBV is most common, for example, in countries with poor sanitation and personal hygiene. So, around 80 per cent of HCCs worldwide occur in East Asia and sub-Saharan Africa. HBV causes 70 per cent of HCCs in Korea, compared with 15 per cent in Japan, and 3 per cent in the USA and Sweden.[1] These figures underscore the importance of taking the precautions outlined in Chapter 4 when travelling to areas where the viruses are common or if you're exposed to other high-risk situations or activities closer to home.

Nevertheless, hepatitis viruses are not the only reason why liver cancer is more widespread in certain parts of the world. For example:

- Aflatoxin is a poison produced by a fungus that grows on mouldy peanuts, wheat, soya, corn, rice and so on, and is especially common in parts of Africa and Asia. However, aflatoxin increases the risk of liver cancer only if people eat food colonized by the fungus over a long time. Indeed, many researchers believe that aflatoxin increases cancer risk only in people infected with HBV.[1]

- Arsenic, which is found in the drinking water of some developing countries, increases the risk of liver cancer.[1]
- Betel quid is prepared from the leaf of a vine, often mixed with areca nut, slaked lime, spices and, sometimes, tobacco. Chewing betel quid as a stimulant and relaxant is relatively common across the Indian subcontinent, Asia and parts of the Pacific. In one study, betel chewing increased the risk of liver cancer around 3.5 times. Furthermore, people infected with HBV who chewed betel were five times more likely to develop liver cancer than those with the virus alone. And chewing betel quid almost doubled the risk of liver cancer in people with HCV.[5]

Diabetes, obesity and liver cancer

In North America, Europe and Japan, HCV and alcohol abuse are the most common causes of HCC. Indeed, HCV can interact with other risk factors, such as NAFLD (page 52) and alcohol abuse, to further increase the likelihood of developing liver cancer.[3]

As mentioned in Chapter 6, obesity can lead to NAFLD, which may help explain why obese people are 2–3 times more likely to develop HCC than their thinner counterparts.[1] Indeed, NASH increases liver cancer risk up to tenfold.[6] Obesity also increases the likelihood that people infected with HBV and HCV will develop HCC. Diabetes makes matters even worse. The risk that a person with diabetes and HBV or HCV will develop HCC is around 100 times higher than in infected people who are neither obese nor diabetic.[1] Incidentally, carrying excess weight is the leading cause of type 2 diabetes (page 54).

Alcohol abuse, smoking and liver cancer

As we saw in Chapter 1, the liver is the body's waste disposal unit and metabolizes alcohol. However, excessive drinking can overwhelm the liver's ability to cope, causing irreparable damage (Chapter 5). So, perhaps not surprisingly, alcohol causes around 5 per cent of avoidable liver cancers in women and 11 per cent in men.[7]

Alcohol seems to increase the risk of liver cancer by triggering cirrhosis, rather than being directly carcinogenic (cancer causing).[1] Nevertheless, in addition to liver cancer, alcohol probably also increases the risk of malignancies of the mouth and throat, oesophagus (food pipe), colon (large bowel), rectum, larynx (voice box) and breast.[7] Chapter 5 offers some suggestions that may help you control your alcohol consumption.

You probably know that smoking is the main cause of lung cancer, accounting for 86 per cent of cases in the UK in 2010. However, smoking can cause several other malignancies, including 65 per cent of cancers in the mouth, throat and oesophagus; 29 per cent of pancreatic cancers; and 22 per cent of stomach cancers. Furthermore, smoking probably caused 27 per cent of liver cancers in men and 15 per cent in women in the UK during 2010.[8] Other investigations suggest that the risk of liver cancer among smokers is even higher. In one study, smoking contributed to almost half (48 per cent) of HCCs, more than chronic HBV (13 per cent), HCV (21 per cent), obesity (16.0 per cent) and heavy alcohol intake (10 per cent).[9]

While estimates of the risk vary, smoking is undoubtedly an important cause of liver cancer. The link makes sense: carcinogens in cigarette smoke can enter the blood through the lungs and trigger cancers in the liver.[4] After all, the liver has an especially rich blood supply. Chapter 11 looks at some ways to quit smoking.

Risk factors you can't control

While you can reduce your chances of catching a hepatitis virus, and you can quit smoking or control your alcohol consumption, there is not much you can do about some risk factors for liver cancer, such as being male, getting older and having a relative who developed the malignancy:

- Around two-thirds (64 per cent) of liver cancers occur in men. In the UK, the lifetime risk for developing liver cancer is 1 in 137 for men and 1 in 244 for women. Differences in risk factors (such as alcohol consumption) probably account for most of the excess risk among men.
- In one study, a family history of liver cancer increased the risk of developing HCC around threefold in men. (The link did not emerge among women).[10]

- The risk of liver cancer rises markedly with advancing age, Cancer Research UK notes: 7 in 10 cases occur in people aged at least 65 years. By contrast, people younger than 50 years of age develop 7 per cent of liver cancers. In part, the increased risk with advancing age reflects the fact that the cancer usually takes many years to emerge after exposure to the carcinogen.
- Having a parent who develops liver cancer increases the risk of developing HCC more than sixfold.[10] This may point to genetic factors influencing the risk, the impact of risk factors you share with other members of your family, or both.
- People with a family history of liver cancer who are infected with HBV or HCV are approximately 72 times more likely to develop HCC than those with neither risk factor.[10]

Although you can do little about, for example, your family history – you can't choose your parents – triggers for liver cancer rarely act in isolation. So, if you quit smoking and reduce your alcohol consumption to safe levels, you'll improve your chances of avoiding liver cancer whether you've contracted a hepatitis virus or have a family history of the malignancy.

Symptoms of liver cancer

Liver cancer often produces vague symptoms that are similar to those typical of other diseases. However, some hints may heighten doctors' suspicions that you've developed liver cancer. For example, a swelling on the right side of your abdomen might arise from a growing cancer. Ascites (page 18) often produce more widespread swelling.

Nevertheless, if you develop any of the symptoms in Table 7.1 you should see your doctor as soon as possible – even if you've already been diagnosed with chronic liver disease. You should also see your doctor, if, for example:

- you have stable cirrhosis and your liver function suddenly worsens;
- you start bleeding into your gut. Watch your stools for changes, such as signs of blood or a black, tar-like consistency;
- you develop ascites.[1]

Table 7.1 Possible symptoms of primary liver cancer

Marked weight loss (such as losing 1 stone if you weigh 11 stone) that cannot be explained (such as by dieting)

Losing your appetite for a few weeks

Vomiting

Feeling full or bloated after eating a relatively small meal

Pain, discomfort or swelling in your tummy (abdomen)

Yellow-tinged skin (jaundice), dark brownish urine, pale clay-coloured faeces

Itching

Sudden worsening of your health if you have chronic hepatitis or cirrhosis

High temperature or sweating

Source: Adapted from Cancer Research UK

Detecting liver cancer

The problems of diagnosing liver cancer based on symptoms alone mean that doctors use a range of techniques to detect the malignancy. However, despite a dramatic improvement in the sensitivity of imaging technology (Chapter 3), doctors rarely detect HCCs that are 1 cm or less in diameter. Biopsy, even guided by sophisticated imaging techniques, could miss such a small target.[3] As this suggests, there is no perfect means to detect liver cancer and doctors will probably use more than one approach.

Blood tests

Apart from performing liver function tests (page 24), doctors may measure levels of a chemical called alpha-fetoprotein in your blood. Normally, only developing foetuses produce alpha-fetoprotein. However, blood levels increase in many people with HCC and some other malignancies. Measuring levels of alpha-fetoprotein can also help doctors assess the effectiveness of treatment: levels fall as the cancer shrinks. Unfortunately, measuring levels of alpha-fetoprotein detects only around 60 per cent of liver cancers.[3]

Imaging

As we saw in Chapter 3, several imaging techniques allow doctors to view your liver in often remarkable detail. So, if you have chronic liver disease, your doctor may suggest regular ultrasound screening.

By looking for changes between visits, ultrasonography can detect around 90 per cent of tumours before symptoms develop.[1] Nevertheless, ultrasonography is more likely to miss tumours that are already present at the first visit because the doctors do not have a previous image for comparison. Overall, ultrasonography can detect around 60–80 per cent of liver cancers.[3] In other cases, doctors may suggest using CT or MRI to detect the cancer.

Biopsy

The definitive way to detect a malignancy is to take a sample and examine the tissue under a microscope for cancer's hallmark changes. However, even biopsies are not infallible and may not detect 30 per cent of HCCs.[3] Furthermore, as mentioned in Chapter 3, in 1–5 per cent of cases the biopsy allows the cancer to spread to another part of the liver.[1] Because of the hazards, when a cancer is larger than 1 cm and you have another risk factor, such as cirrhosis, doctors may diagnose HCC using imaging alone.[1] So, it's important to discuss the advantages and disadvantages of the various techniques fully with your doctor.

Treating liver cancer

As we have seen, just 5 per cent of people with liver cancer live for at least 5 years after their diagnosis. This is a particularly bleak prognosis; for instance, 85 per cent of women with breast cancer and 81 per cent of men with prostate cancer in England are alive 5 years after diagnosis. Despite this poor outlook, provided doctors detect the malignancy early enough, surgery and liver transplantation cure some hepatic cancers. Various drugs and surgery can lengthen your survival, even if a cure is impossible.[3] That's why it's important to see your doctor as soon as possible if you think there is anything wrong.

Surgery to remove the cancer

Surgery to cut away the cancer (hepatic resection) is the treatment of choice for HCC if you're one of the 5 per cent or so of people who develop the cancer without marked cirrhosis. However, surgeons need to balance the risks and benefits for each person who has developed cirrhosis. In these people, resection can result in liver

failure.[3] And as we saw when we looked at the Child–Pugh classification (page 26), the likelihood of death after major surgery rises
dramatically as liver damage worsens.

Around 1 in 6 people (15 per cent) live for at least 5 years after
surgery to remove liver cancer. However, the outlook depends on
the size of the cancer. More than half of patients with tumours
less than 3 cm across live at least 5 years after the operation.
Unfortunately, Cancer Research UK points out, doctors diagnose
only about 1 in 10 liver cancers in the early stages when surgery can
still markedly improve chances of survival.

Surgeons tend to use resection for patients with a single tumour.
Other approaches, such as transplantation, ablation or chemoembolization (see below), might be more appropriate when the liver
contains more than one tumour. The more cancers you have in
your liver, the greater the risk of recurrence. A full and frank discussion of the risks and benefits can help you decide the best approach
for you.

Liver transplant

Liver transplants transformed HCC treatment by raising the prospect of a cure and resolving the underlying cirrhosis.[3] Indeed, 80
per cent of recipients are still alive at least 4 years after receiving
their new organ, according to Cancer Research UK.

One study, for example, included people with a single HCC of 5
cm or smaller, or up to three malignancies each of which was 3 cm
or smaller that had not spread into the blood vessels or outside the
liver. Three-quarters of these patients were still alive 4 years after
their transplant. Just 15 per cent of the cancers recurred.[3] However,
there are too few donated organs to meet demand and you'll need
to take powerful drugs (immunosuppressants) to reduce the risk
that you'll reject your new liver. Unfortunately, immunosuppressants can cause potentially serious side effects (page 20).

Ablation

Doctors may try to destroy early HCC by injecting a chemical (such
as ethanol or acetic acid) into the cancer guided by imaging – a tech-
nique called ablation. Other ablation techniques use radio waves,
microwaves or lasers to heat the tissue, or extreme cold (cryoabla-
tion), to destroy cancerous cells.[3]

For example, ablation using ethanol and radio waves can destroy almost all HCCs that are smaller than 2 cm. However, ablation is less effective against larger cancers. So, generally, surgeons do not use ablation to treat tumours larger than 5 cm. Furthermore, ablation is not suitable for cancers near major blood vessels, bile ducts, the bowel, heart or other critical organs: the risk of collateral damage to the healthy tissue is too high. But for selected patients, the chances of surviving 5 years after ablation are about the same as those following surgery: for example, 50–75 per cent of patients with Child–Pugh A cirrhosis (page 26).[3]

Chemoembolization

You've probably heard of deep vein thrombosis – when a blood clot develops inside a vein, usually in the leg, when you're immobilized (such as during a long-haul flight). Fragments of the clot can break off and travel through the bloodstream and lodge in smaller vessels supplying the brain, lung or another organ, causing a stroke or a life-threatening lung condition called a pulmonary embolism. The blockage starves the brain or lung of oxygen and so the cells die.

Once a cancer is bigger than about 1–2 mm, the tumour is too large to absorb oxygen and nutrients directly from the surrounding tissue. So, the tumour produces chemicals that stimulate the development of new blood vessels (a process known as angiogenesis) to fuel the cancer's continuing growth. Blocking these blood vessels will starve the cancer of oxygen and nutrients and so limit growth. Indeed, some drugs for liver and several other cancers work by reducing angiogenesis.

Doctors treat certain liver cancers by blocking the cancer's blood supply (embolization) by, for example, using tiny spheres. In addition, the spheres slowly release a cancer drug – attacking the malignancy on two fronts. More than half of patients show 'extensive' death of cancerous tissue following chemoembolization. On average, carefully selected patients treated with the most advanced forms of chemoembolization combined with chemotherapy survive around 3 years. However, cancers can develop other new blood vessels that bypass the block. And chemoembolization does not attack small cancers that have not yet produced blood vessels, but which could develop into large tumours. As a result, oncologists tend to reserve chemoembolization for large cancers or numerous malignancies that are unsuitable for surgery.[3]

Drugs for liver cancer

Until recently, doctors did not have an effective drug for patients with advanced liver cancer. However, a growing number of drugs are showing promise. One of these, called sorafenib, blocks some key signalling pathways inside a cell that lead to cancer growth and promote the formation of new blood vessels.

In one study, patients with advanced cancer taking sorafenib survived for, on average, 10.7 months compared with 7.9 months in those taking an inactive placebo. The cancer progressed after, on average, 5.5 months in patients taking sorafenib and 2.8 months in those receiving placebo.[3]

Our rapidly advancing understanding of liver cancer's causes, development and spread means that other drugs will probably reach the clinic over the next few years. You could ask your oncologist whether you would benefit from taking part in a clinical study of a new treatment for liver cancer.

Prevention is better than cure

Clearly, however, prevention is better than treatment. So, follow the advice about smoking cessation, controlling alcohol consumption and avoiding infection. Make sure your jabs are up to date: vaccination can prevent HCC linked to HBV, for example.[3] And if you're chronically infected with hepatitis viruses, using interferon and antivirals should prevent progression of liver disease and, possibly, reduce HCC risk. However, antivirals are less effective at preventing HCC once you develop cirrhosis.[3]

HCC is usually the last stage in the development of liver disease that began many years previously with an infection, excessive drinking or smoking. In many cases, the cancer develops because of the extensive scarring caused by these risk factors. So, you can reduce your likelihood of developing the malignancy – even if you already have chronic liver disease – by lifestyle measures such as avoiding alcohol, quitting smoking and ensuring you attend your screening appointments. Early detection and liver transplantation are usually the only realistic prospects of curing this all too often deadly malignancy.

8

Other diseases of the liver

Alcohol abuse, viruses and obesity cause most liver diseases. However, more than 100 ailments can damage the liver. There is not space to look at all of these here. But the following examples illustrate the wide range of conditions that potentially undermine the health of this critical organ.

For example, as mentioned in Chapter 3, antibodies detect and help destroy invading bacteria, viruses and parasites, and also mop up damaged or cancerous cells. When antibodies attack the liver and gall bladder, patients may develop, depending on the cells affected, primary sclerosing cholangitis, primary biliary cirrhosis or autoimmune hepatitis.

In other cases, patients inherit abnormal genes from their parents that result in liver damage. For instance, some people have a faulty gene that means they accumulate excessive levels of iron (haemochromatosis) or copper (Wilson's disease) in several tissues, including the liver. Other genetic changes mean that patients produce inadequate levels of a key enzyme (page 74) called alpha-1 antitrypsin.

In addition, numerous chemicals, including some widely used medicines, can irreparably poison the liver. Indeed, paracetamol is the most common cause of acute (rapid-onset) liver failure in the UK.[1] But in many cases, doctors cannot identify a cause for the hepatic damage, so-called cryptogenic liver disease. The National Digestive Diseases Information Clearinghouse (<http://digestive. niddk.nih.gov>) and The British Liver Trust (<www.britishlivertrust. org.uk>) are excellent sources of information about the myriad forms of liver disease.

Porphyria

How would you react if your urine turned purple? Normally, a biological pigment called urochrome is responsible for urine's yellow colour. However, in some cases of porphyria the body excretes large amounts of proteins called porphyrins in the urine. The high porphyrin levels can give urine a red or purple colour. Indeed, the term porphyria comes from the Greek for purple. However, porphyria is not a single disease.

The body converts a chemical called aminolevulinic acid to haem, the red pigment in blood, in seven steps, each controlled by a different enzyme. The British Porphyria Association (BPA) explains that porphyria arises when a faulty gene means that one of the enzymes in the chain does not work properly. As the enzyme does not convert the chemical to the next step, levels of the preceding protein rise – causing the condition's often debilitating symptoms. In addition to abnormal genes, heavy alcohol consumption, iron supplements, certain drugs and liver infections can trigger a form of the disease called porphyria cutanea tarda. The seven subtypes of porphyria differ in their symptoms and outlook – and some are very rare. So, this section introduces the disease. If you want to know more contact the BPA.

Acute attacks

According to the BPA, four types of porphyria cause acute attacks, of which acute intermittent porphyria and variegate porphyria are the most common. Fortunately, only about 1 in 5 people with the gene for one of these porphyrias develops sudden (also called acute) attacks, which are characterized by:

- severe pain in the stomach, back or thighs;
- nausea, vomiting and constipation;
- red, brown or purple urine (the sample can initially look normal, but changes colour when stored);
- low levels of salt or sodium (page 83) in the blood;
- rapid pulse and dangerously high blood pressure (hypertension);
- loss of movement in the arms or legs. While uncommon, the BPA comments, loss of movement can emerge several weeks after the acute attack.

These symptoms seem to emerge when the level of one of two chemicals (aminolevulinic acid and porphobilinogen) in the pathway that makes haem exceeds the safe level and starts damaging nerves. Some people experience only one or two acute attacks, which may be triggered by, for example, alcohol and certain drugs. You can think of the genetic disease forming the soil: the trigger factor is the seed that allows the porphyria to emerge.

Skin symptoms

Porphyrins, which are light-sensitive, can accumulate in the skin. So, when light hits skin laden with porphyrins, the reaction damages the surrounding tissues. As a result, the BPA points out, the skin of people with one of five forms of porphyria (such as congenital erythropoietic porphyria) can blister, burn easily in the sun and, in some cases, scar.

Porphyria cutanea tarda is the most common cause of porphyria's skin symptoms. Hereditary coproporphyria and variegate porphyria can cause both acute attacks and skin symptoms. The other forms of cutaneous porphyria cause only skin symptoms. Treatment largely focuses on avoiding trigger factors (such as sun exposure and certain medicines) and so depends on which type of porphyria you suffer from. Contact the BPA or your doctor for more information.

Haemochromatosis

Iron is essential for red blood cells to carry oxygen and for several other critical biochemical reactions. However, you can have too much of a good thing. Iron overload, called haemochromatosis, occurs when the body stores too much iron.

People with hereditary (primary) haemochromatosis are born with a genetic defect that leads to excessive levels of iron accumulating in several places around their body, including the liver. Patients with alcoholic liver disease, NASH or HCV infection also have a tendency towards accumulating iron – so-called secondary haemochromatosis. Indeed, up to 30 per cent of people with liver disease have excessive levels of iron in their blood. About 10 per cent have high iron levels in their liver.[2]

It might sound a tad medieval, but doctors treat haemochromatosis by draining blood (phlebotomy). Initially, doctors drain 500 ml (about a pint – the same as a blood donation) every week until levels normalize. But this can take a year. They will then remove blood every 2–4 weeks to keep iron at safe levels. If phlebotomy is not appropriate, doctors may use a drug called deferasirox, which removes iron from blood.

Wilson's disease

In addition to iron, the body needs small amounts of zinc, sodium, potassium and copper. Again, some people accumulate excessive levels of these essential elements. We'll look at ways to reduce levels of sodium when we consider salt in Chapter 9. And about 1 in 40,000 people develop Wilson's disease, a genetic disorder that prevents the body from removing copper it does not need. So, levels rise in the liver, brain, eyes and other organs, potentially causing life-threatening damage.

People with Wilson's disease inherit two abnormal copies of a gene called *ATP7B*. This disease is 'recessive'. In other words, if you have one abnormal gene and one normal gene you will not develop the symptoms (but you can pass the abnormal gene on to your children). As a result, most people with Wilson's disease don't know anyone else in their family with the disease. In general, symptoms appear between 5 and 35 years of age. However, the disease can emerge at any time between 2 and 72 years of age.

Symptoms of Wilson's disease

Normally, the liver stores small amounts of copper and excretes the excess in bile. Once the liver stores are filled, the excess copper remains in the organs, initially attacking the liver, the central nervous system (brain and spinal cord), or both. In some cases, the patient rapidly develops liver failure. However, most patients develop signs and symptoms of chronic liver disease, including jaundice, fluid in the legs (oedema) or abdomen (ascites), easy bruising and fatigue. Furthermore, the build-up of copper in the brain and spinal cord can cause:

- problems with speech, swallowing and physical coordination
- tremors or uncontrolled movements
- muscle stiffness
- altered behaviour.

Meanwhile, copper deposits in other organs can cause, for example, anaemia, low levels of white blood cells, slow blood clotting, osteoporosis (brittle bone disease), arthritis and characteristic 'Kayser–Fleischer rings' (the accumulation of copper in the eyes creates a rusty-brown ring around the iris and the rim of the cornea).

Treating Wilson's disease

Treatment aims to remove excess copper, reduce copper intake and treat any liver or central nervous system damage. For example:

- The drugs d-penicillamine and trientine hydrochloride release stores of copper from organs into the bloodstream; the copper is then excreted. The surge in copper can initially make the symptoms worse, although liver function, physical and mental symptoms often improve if patients continue treatment.
- Another group of medicines, zinc acetate and other zinc salts, do not remove copper rapidly enough to treat symptoms. However, regularly taking zinc salts blocks absorption of copper from food.
- People with Wilson's disease need to control their consumption of foods rich in copper by avoiding shellfish or liver and eating mushrooms, broccoli, nuts and chocolate in moderation once symptoms abate.

Alpha-1 antitrypsin deficiency

Alpha-1 antitrypsin (A1AT) deficiency is another inherited condition. But this time, patients lack A1AT, a protein made by the liver. Some people produce low levels of A1AT, which does not work properly. Most cases are mild and never cause symptoms, especially if patients don't smoke (see below).

A1AT has various roles. In the lungs, for example, A1AT mops up an enzyme called neutrophil elastase, which normally destroys damaged or old lung cells, foreign particles and bacteria. A1AT prevents neutrophil elastase from damaging healthy lung tissue. So, in A1AT deficiency, the high levels of neutrophil elastase cause a potentially debilitating condition called emphysema, which typically emerges in people over 50 years old. However, smoking is a far more common cause of emphysema than A1AT deficiency.

A1AT deficiency also contributes to liver disease. For example, some newborn babies with A1AT deficiency show signs of hepatic disease, such as jaundice, clay-coloured stools, excessive bleeding or an enlarged liver. This neonatal hepatitis syndrome usually emerges between 4 days and 6 weeks after birth. Most affected babies get better, although occasionally a newborn baby rapidly develops liver

Emphysema

After passing through the nose and mouth, air flows along the trachea, which is about 10–16 cm long and about 2 cm wide. The trachea forks into two major bronchi, one to each lung. Each major bronchus divides another 10 to 25 times into bronchi and then bronchioles, which end in 300–500 million alveoli. Each alveolus, which looks like a cauliflower floret, is about 0.1–0.2 mm in diameter. The bronchial tree's shape packs a vast area into a relatively small volume: our lungs contain approximately 1,500 miles of airways. In an adult, the surface area of the alveoli is about 70 m², roughly the same as a singles tennis court. A network of around 620 miles of capillaries (small, thin blood vessels) surrounds the alveoli. Oxygen dissolves in the fluid covering the thin alveoli and crosses into the bloodstream. Red blood cells pick up and carry oxygen to tissues throughout your body.

Alveoli and small airways depend on the support of the surrounding tissues to remain open. Emphysema destroys this support. That's one reason why the airways of people with emphysema become obstructed and collapse when they exhale. This traps air, which can stretch the lungs and makes breathing much more difficult. As emphysema progresses, the alveoli form large, irregular pockets with holes in their walls. Not surprisingly, these changes hinder the transfer of carbon dioxide and oxygen. So people with emphysema cough, wheeze, feel breathless and are vulnerable to lung infections.

failure. Liver disease due to A1AT deficiency can also emerge in later life. So, people with A1AT deficiency should:

- not drink alcohol and, when possible, avoid medicines that may harm the liver (page 79);
- like the rest of us, eat a diet with plenty of fresh fruit and vegetables, an issue we'll return to in Chapter 9;
- take exercise to help boost the immune system;
- avoid tobacco smoke and pollution. A1AT-deficient lungs are especially vulnerable to damage by pollution and smoking. As a result, people with A1AT deficiency (and those around them) should quit smoking (page 113).

Autoimmune diseases

Autoimmune hepatitis follows an attack on liver cells by the body's immune system, marshalled by antibodies that incorrectly regard healthy cells as 'foreign' proteins. Almost any tissue can face an autoimmune attack, including muscles, kidneys and the liver. Typically, an autoimmune attack causes inflammation and, over time, damages the tissue.

Indeed, autoimmune hepatitis is often relatively serious and, if not treated, can end in cirrhosis and liver failure. (Doctors treat autoimmune hepatitis with drugs such as steroids and azathioprine, which dampen the immune response.) And this immunological civil war can cause other autoimmune conditions affecting the liver and gall bladder.

Primary biliary cirrhosis

During primary biliary cirrhosis (PBC), an autoimmune attack slowly destroys bile ducts. Bile leaks from the ducts damage the surrounding liver cells. As the liver can compensate for often quite extensive damage, PBC may not cause symptoms. But in other cases, over many years, the damage from the bile causes cirrhosis.

According to the PBC Foundation, up to 1 in 1,000 women in high-risk areas such as north-east England and Scotland develop PBC, although many don't develop symptoms. Nine women develop PBC for every man with the disease. The condition tends to emerge between the ages of 30 and 55 years.

The trigger for the autoimmune attack is usually unknown. However, a few clues have emerged. For example, some patients have a close relative with the disease, suggesting a genetic link. Furthermore, PBC may emerge during or following pregnancy. Some infections, toxins and stress may also trigger the autoimmune assault on the liver cells.

Drugs such as ursodeoxycholic acid and medicines that reduce inflammation can help treat PBC. Occasionally, people with PBC need a liver transplant. In addition, many people find that they need to adapt their lifestyle to cope with the fatigue that many people with PBC endure. The PBC Foundation adds that eating regular small meals often ensures that bile has some food to digest, which helps spare your liver.

Primary sclerosing cholangitis

In primary sclerosing cholangitis (PSC), scar tissue narrows and then completely blocks the bile ducts, preventing the normal flow of bile out of the liver. The resulting hepatic damage causes the typical symptoms of liver disease (such as itching, jaundice and abdominal pain) and, in some patients, leads to cirrhosis, portal hypertension and liver failure. The cause of PSC is not clear. However, an autoimmune attack probably contributes to the damage.

Around twice as many men as women develop PSC. However, some people with PSC haven't developed symptoms when they are diagnosed. And the speed of progression of PSC, severity and the symptoms vary widely. Currently, there is no cure or treatment to slow progression and some people eventually need liver transplants.

Gall stones

Gall stones are pebble-like deposits inside the gall bladder, which range in size from a grain of sand to a golf ball. Cholesterol excreted in the bile makes up most stones. Less commonly, high levels of bilirubin, released during the destruction of old red blood cells, forms 'pigment' stones.

Several factors may increase the risk of developing gall stones, which are listed in Table 8.1.

Many people are unaware that they have gall stones: doctors diagnose the problem on an X-ray, during surgery and so on. However, large stones blocking the bile duct (choledocholithiasis) can cause pain in the middle to right upper abdomen (biliary colic). The pain may be excruciating, sharp, cramping, or dull and may spread to the back or below the right shoulder blade. Biliary colic fades if the stone passes into the duodenum. Other people develop fever, jaundice, pass clay-coloured stools, or experience nausea and vomiting. See your GP if you develop any of these symptoms.

Table 8.1 Factors that may increase the risk of developing gall stones

Factor	Explanation
Being female	Oestrogen from pregnancy, hormone replacement therapy and the Pill seem to increase the risk. Overall, two women develop gall stones for each man with the condition.
Diabetes	People with diabetes often show high levels of triglycerides (page 8), which increases the likelihood of developing gall stones.
Genetics	Gall stones seem to run in families.
Weight	Even being moderately overweight seems to increase the risk. The link between obesity and gall stones seems to be especially strong in women. Chapter 9 looks at some ways to help you lose weight. But avoid rapid weight loss ('crash diets'), which can increase your risk of developing gall stones.
Unhealthy diet	A diet high in fat and cholesterol and low in fibre increases the amount of cholesterol in bile and can stop the gall bladder from emptying properly.
Age	You are more likely to develop gall stones once you are over 60 years of age.
Cholesterol-lowering drugs	These may increase the amount removed in the bile (see Unhealthy diet above).

Source: Adapted from National Digestive Diseases Information Clearinghouse

Treating gall stones

Usually, gall stones that don't cause symptoms do not need surgery. However, people who develop symptoms will need surgery to remove their gall bladder as soon as possible. Traditionally, doctors removed the gall bladder through one large incision in the patient's abdomen (a procedure called open cholecystectomy). The modern procedure (laparoscopic cholecystectomy) removes the gall bladder through a series of smaller cuts, which speeds recovery and is less likely to cause complications.

Doctors can also prescribe certain medicines (chenodeoxycholic acid or ursodeoxycholic acid) to dissolve gall stones made from cholesterol. However, these may take 2 years or more to work. Another approach uses sound waves (electrohydraulic or extracorporeal shock wave lithotripsy) to break up the stones. Doctors tend to use shock wave lithotripsy when patients cannot have surgery. However, in both cases, gall stones may form again when treatment ends.

Medicines that harm the liver

As mentioned in Chapter 1, the liver is the body's main waste disposal unit, breaking down many medicines and a range of other chemicals. Usually, the liver makes the medicine less active. But some drugs do not work unless they are first converted by the liver – so-called prodrugs. Furthermore, the way the liver metabolizes certain drugs can lead to potentially serious interactions.

Activating drugs

Several painkillers contain codeine, such as co-codamol, which also includes paracetamol. Codeine itself is not very effective. However, enzymes in your liver convert between 5 and 15 per cent of a dose of codeine into morphine, which alleviates the pain. However, up to 10 per cent of people of European descent lack the enzyme that converts codeine to morphine. So these people find that codeine does not work.

Some drugs trigger the liver to produce larger quantities of one or more cytochrome P450 enzymes (page 6) – so-called inducers. If you take the inducer with another drug broken down by same enzyme, the liver may remove the second drug too quickly. And the medicine may then not alleviate the disease it was prescribed to treat. For example, St John's wort (*Hypericum perforatum*), a herbal antidepressant, potently induces one of these enzymes – CYP3A4. So if you take a drug metabolized by CYP3A4 with St John's wort, the medicine may not work as well as it should.

Taking a drug metabolized by CYP3A4 along with a medicine (or even grapefruit juice) that inhibits the same enzyme could allow blood levels of the first medicine to rise, potentially causing serious side effects. Several drugs inhibit CYP3A4, including a group of antibiotics called macrolides (which includes erythromycin) and some calcium-channel blockers, used to treat, for example, hypertension and angina. Furthermore, CYP3A4 metabolizes several statins – notably simvastatin and atorvastatin – used to lower levels of cholesterol in the blood and so reduce the risk of heart disease. Taking some statins with drugs that inhibit CYP3A4 could elevate concentrations of statins, potentially damaging your muscles and causing other side effects.[3]

The risk of interactions is one reason why you should let your doctor and pharmacist know when you are using herbal remedies (page 103) and other medicines that you've been prescribed or you've bought over the counter.

Nevertheless, in research performed during 2008, 30 per cent of people in the UK prescribed a statin metabolized by CYP3A4 also received a drug that researchers had shown in scientific studies inhibited the cytochrome.[3] It is impossible for doctors to keep up to date with every scientific study that might influence practice. Worryingly, however, 11 per cent of people prescribed a statin metabolized by CYP3A4 received a drug highlighted as inhibiting this cytochrome by the Medicines and Healthcare products Regulatory Agency (MHRA), which regulates drugs in the UK, or by the detailed information on a drug – the Summary of Product Characteristics (SPC).[3] So it's important to double check the SPC (<www.medicines.org.uk/emc>), which will warn you about potential interactions with foods and other drugs. If you're worried speak to your pharmacist.

Furthermore, because scarring destroys cells that break down toxins, chronic liver disease can undermine hepatic function and, in turn, the body's ability to metabolize certain drugs. This can lead to high blood levels and, as a result, side effects. At doses prescribed by your doctor, most drugs are safe, despite the altered metabolism and liver function. However, in some cases, your doctor will lower the dose to compensate for the fraction of drug no longer removed by the liver. Again, check the SPC or speak to your pharmacist.

Drugs and chronic liver disease

As a rule, people with chronic liver disease should avoid taking drugs that could further damage hepatocytes – especially because the cells responsible for metabolizing potential toxins receive a higher level of potentially harmful chemicals and lack some of the defences other parts of the liver use to prevent hepatotoxicity. So, hepatocytes that metabolize drugs are also particularly susceptible to hazardous chemicals.[4]

However, numerous drugs are hepatotoxic, including some medicines used to lower cholesterol, certain antifungals and several painkillers. For example, almost everyone takes non-steroidal anti-inflammatory drugs (NSAIDS), such as ibuprofen, aspirin and diclofenac, to alleviate pain and inflammation. In a few people infected with HCV, ibuprofen increases levels of enzymes included in liver function tests more than 20-fold. Unfortunately, doctors cannot predict who will develop liver damage when they take NSAIDs.[2] So, people with chronic liver disease should avoid NSAIDS, unless advised otherwise by their doctor.

Paracetamol is not strictly an NSAID, but it causes hepatotoxicity. And the higher the dose of paracetamol, the greater the risk of liver damage. In some cases, less than 4 g paracetamol a day can cause hepatotoxicity, usually when the person is severely malnourished or has drunk alcohol.[2] Indeed, in 2010, paracetamol poisoning contributed to 199 deaths – in other words, the death certificate mentions the painkiller. That's more than the number who died from cocaine (mentioned on 144 death certificates), amphetamines (56) or cannabis (11). So if you have liver disease, don't buy pain-killers from a supermarket or pharmacy without checking with a pharmacist or doctor first.

As people with chronic liver disease may be less able to tolerate hepatotoxicity when it occurs, your doctor may suggest liver function tests (page 24) before you start taking a medicine and perform the tests regularly during treatment. They may decide to stop treatment if levels of the liver enzymes rise excessively. You should tell your doctor if you develop symptoms that might indicate hepatotoxicity, such as jaundice, weight loss, nausea, itching, fatigue and pain in the right upper abdomen.[2]

9

Diet and liver disease

Humans did not evolve to chomp on junk food high in sugar and fat, and low in essential nutrients. Rather than sweets, cakes, pastries, takeaway food, ready meals and so on, we evolved to eat, essentially, a hunter–gatherer diet that is rich in complex carbohydrates (such as starch from fruit and vegetables) and low in animal fats. Our hunter–gatherer ancestors also kept moving in their search for food and water. Inevitably, most modern-day hunter–gatherers are physically fit and relatively lean. In addition, a healthy diet can boost your immune responses, may help your liver heal and mop up tissue-damaging free radicals (page 56).

By contrast, the typical modern Western diet produces an overabundance of energy. If you do not burn this energy off, the body stores the surplus in fat cells as a precaution against famine. But in industrialized nations we can easily access food. So, we never use these stores. As a result we gain weight, especially around our middle (central obesity). This contributes to the risk of developing numerous diseases, including heart attacks, diabetes and NAFLD.

So everyone, but especially people with liver disease or another chronic condition, needs to ensure that they eat a healthy, balanced diet. Changing your diet can seem daunting. But many people find that it takes only a month or so of eating – or not eating – a food to form a habit. Indeed, some people (myself among them) who switch to skimmed milk soon find that they dislike the taste of full-fat milk. And many people find they soon lose their sweet tooth or do not need as much salt.

A healthy diet is also one of the best ways to detox. As we'll see in Chapter 10, many doctors are cynical about the benefits of detox. However, most complementary healers emphasize the importance of a healthy diet as a cornerstone of detox. And everyone agrees that a healthy diet is one of the best ways to bolster your health and well-being. So, go through your kitchen cupboards, fridge and freezer and get rid of all the processed, refined, fat- and salt-laden food. And go to your local library or surf around the Internet and try to become more creative in the kitchen. A healthy diet does not need to be boring.

Salt

People who develop cirrhosis tend to retain too much salt in their blood. So, your doctor may suggest restricting the amount of salt you eat.[1] However, it's a lesson that almost every one of us, whether or not we have chronic liver disease, could learn: many people in the UK eat too much salt, increasing their risk of several diseases.

High levels of salt (sodium chloride) in your blood can damage your cells. So, your body retains fluid to dilute the high levels of salt. But retaining fluid increases your blood pressure. That means that a high salt intake makes it more likely you'll develop hypertension, which can lead to strokes and heart disease. Despite the risks, the British Dietetic Association (BDA) comments that the average UK adult eats around 8.6 g of salt a day – that's about two teaspoons. The recommended intake for healthy adults is 6 g of salt a day. But you should follow your doctor's advice: some people with liver disease and certain other conditions (e.g. heart failure and hypertension) need to consume even less.

It's easy to tell that some snacks are salty. But many foods contain 'hidden' salt, so your taste buds will not set the alarm bells ringing. For example, food manufacturers add surprisingly large amounts of salt to some soups, bread, biscuits and breakfast cereals. Indeed, salt already added to food accounts for three-quarters of our daily consumption.

Easy ways to cut your salt intake

- Avoid foods that are high in salt (such as smoked meat and fish).
- Add as little salt as you can during baking and cooking.
- Banish the salt cellar from the table.
- Ask restaurants and takeaways for no salt.
- Check levels of added salt and fat in self-basting poultry.
- Look for low-salt ketchup, pickles, mustard, yeast extract, stock cubes and so on.
- Try using herbs, spices, chopped chillies and lime or lemon juice to give grains and other bland foods more taste.

Table 9.1 Salt levels in food

Level	Salt content (g per 100 g)	Sodium content (g per 100 g)
High	More than 1.5	More than 0.6
Medium	0.3–1.5	0.1–0.6
Low	0.3 or less	0.1 or less

Source: Adapted from the British Dietetic Association

So, always read the label and try to stick to low-salt (Table 9.1) foods. The BDA advises choosing meals and sandwiches with less than 0.5 g sodium (1.25 g salt) per meal. Choose individual foods, such as soups and sauces, with less than 0.3 g sodium (0.75 g) per serving. Some labels list sodium, rather than salt. Chemically, table salt is sodium chloride. To convert sodium to salt, multiply by 2.5. So, 0.4 g of sodium is 1 g of salt. You can convert salt to sodium by dividing by 2.5.

Fighting the fat

Some of us (myself from time to time if I'm honest) lament the end of going to work fuelled by a fry-up. In 1989 we ate, on average, 112 g of fat a day, the British Heart Foundation remarks. By 2008 our fat intake had declined to 83 g a day. Yet many of us still eat too much fat – one reason why the nation's waistbands are bulging. Fat is the most concentrated source of energy in our diet: 1 g provides 9 calories. So, reducing fat aids weight reduction, helps you avoid heart disease and type 2 diabetes (page 56), and reduces the risk of NAFLD – quite apart from the other health benefits.

A diet high in fat, especially from animal sources, boosts levels of cholesterol in your blood, which increases your risk of developing gall stones (page 77), heart attacks and some strokes. But despite its bad press, cholesterol is essential for health and well-being. For example, cholesterol:

- is a key part of the membranes that surround every cell;
- is a component of the myelin sheath that envelops certain types of nerve and ensures signals travel properly;
- forms the backbone of several hormones, including oestrogen, testosterone and progesterone.

But poor diets and a lack of exercise (which burns up fat) mean that many of us have too much of a good thing.

Types of fat

Broadly, foods contain two types of fat:

- Saturated fat comes mainly from animal sources, and is generally solid at room temperature.
- Unsaturated fat derives mainly from vegetables, nuts and seeds, and is usually liquid at room temperature. Olive oil is an unsaturated fat, for example. There are two main subtypes: monounsaturated and polyunsaturated. As we'll see, fish is especially high in a particularly beneficial polyunsaturated fat (page 88).

Controlling cholesterol

The amount of cholesterol in your blood depends more on the amount of saturated fat – the animal fat in meat, full-fat dairy products, cakes, biscuits, pastries and so on – you eat than the amount of cholesterol in your diet. Indeed, few foods, with the notable exceptions of eggs, kidneys, prawns and liver, contain high levels of cholesterol. As a result, diet accounts for only around one-third of the cholesterol in our bodies.

Indeed, the traditional advice that you need to eat no more than three eggs a week is now outdated. Indeed, eggs are one the most nutritious foods, which makes sense when you think how well they support growth. For example, eggs are rich in protein (see below) and a great source of vitamins A, B, D and E as well as zinc, iron and other minerals. As we've seen, antioxidant vitamins mop up the free radicals that may contribute to liver disease, while vitamin E helps NASH (page 55).

Rather than worrying about cholesterol, focus on saturated fat. As we've seen, the liver converts saturated fat into cholesterol. Eating foods rich in saturated fat also slows the rate at which your body removes cholesterol. However, the BDA notes that most people in the UK eat about 20 per cent more than the recommended levels of saturated fat for the general population (no more than 20 g for women and 30g for men a day).

So, most of us should try to eat less saturated fat and more low-fat foods. Avoid high-fat foods, which the BDA defines as containing more than 5 g of saturated fat per 100 g. Try to eat more low-fat foods, in other words those containing 1.5 g or less saturated fat per 100 g. Table 9.2 suggests some ways you could cut your consumption of saturated fat.

Table 9.2 Foods high in saturated fat and some alternatives

	Avoid	Lower saturated fat alternative
Snacks	Crisps/savoury snacks cooked in oil	Fresh or dried fruit, handful of nuts
Fats for cooking and spreading	Lard, dripping, ghee, cream and butter	Olive, sunflower, soya or rapeseed (blended vegetable) oils, margarines and spreads
Meat	Processed varieties: sausages, burgers, pâté, salami, meat pies and pasties	Lean cuts of meat and mince (check labels or ask the butcher) Trim off as much fat as you can or ask the butcher to remove the fat Skinless chicken and turkey Vegetarian options (lentils, chick peas and soya) Try Vegemince or soya mince instead of ground beef; if you find the taste a little bland add chillies, spices and herbs
Fish	Deep-fried (e.g. takeaway) fish and chips	Oily fish (page 88), especially grilled or baked; bake fish in the 'foil' packets you can buy from some supermarkets
Sauces	Creamy or cheesy sauces	Tomato- or vegetable-based sauces (ideally, make your own – it's easy!)
Dairy	Full-fat varieties	Skimmed (or at least semi-skimmed) milk; reduced-fat cheddar and low-fat yoghurt Grate cheese or use a strongly flavoured variety, which may mean you need to use less
Cooking	Pan or deep fry	Grill, steam or oven bake Avoid breadcrumbs that soak up fat

Source: Adapted from the British Dietetic Association

Protein

Protein's numerous essential biological roles include:

- helping the liver and other tissues repair and regenerate;
- forming specialized proteins, such as enzymes that speed up the chemical reactions that are essential for life;
- forming the scaffold that supports the cell's shape;
- making antibodies, which are essential for fighting infections.

So, unless your doctor tells you otherwise eat a 'healthy' amount of protein: the BDA suggests that the 'general sedentary population' should eat between 0.80 and 1.0 g of protein per kg of your body-weight each day. Endurance athletes (1.2–1.4 g per kg bodyweight) and strength athletes need slightly more (1.2–1.7 g per kg body-weight). However, a liver damaged by, for example, cirrhosis may not use protein effectively, potentially leading to muscle wasting and increasing the risk of osteoporosis (page 15). As a result, people with liver disease may need to eat plenty of protein, such as 1.0–1.5 g a day for each kg of bodyweight.[1]

While eating sufficient protein is essential for good health, it's important to get the balance right. For example, a high intake of protein seems to increase the risk of colon cancer. So, the government recommends that healthy adults should not eat more than twice the recommended protein level. Furthermore, people who eat large amounts of red meat may be between 24 and 36 per cent more likely to develop diabetes, which, as we've seen, is intimately linked to NAFLD. And it's the protein, rather than just saturated fat, that's to blame.[2]

Protein sources include chicken, turkey, fish, beans and legumes. However, animal protein such as meat, chicken and fish can be loaded with saturated fat. So, choose the leanest cuts of meat and trim any visible fat. That's one reason why chicken helps you control your fat consumption. Most of the fat is outside the muscle, so it's easily removed. The rest of your protein intake should come from, for example, soya products, yoghurt, nuts, seeds, legumes and fish. Indeed, eating some fish offers other benefits, as we'll see now.

Fish and omega-3 fatty acids

Life inside the Arctic Circle is tough. Few plants survive. So, the traditional diet of First Nation Arctic people consists almost entirely of fish, seal and other meats. In the 1970s, for example, Greenland Inuit people ate around 400 g of seafood a day.[3] Despite this meat-based diet, First Nation Arctic people seem to be less vulnerable to several diseases, including diabetes, heart disease, arthritis and asthma, than people in industrialized countries.

But, like all of us, people in the Arctic are what they eat. Traditional diets of First Nation Arctic people are packed with fish and animals that, in turn, eat marine life. So, Inuits eat large amounts of polyunsaturated fish oils (called n-3, or omega-3, poly-unsaturated fatty acids; PUFAs) that have several important health benefits including:

- reducing inflammation (which as we've seen increases in many liver diseases);
- boosting levels of the healthy fat (HDL) in blood;
- cutting triglyceride levels (a leading cause of steatosis and heart disease);
- lowering dangerously raised blood pressure (hypertension), which is also linked to some liver diseases;
- reducing steatosis, countering insulin resistance (page 57) and lowering inflammation in the liver.[4]

Many of these observations emerged from animal and experimental studies. In general, investigations in humans support these findings, although scientists believe that further studies need to confirm the benefits on the liver.[4] But there is little doubt that fish oils can markedly reduce triglyceride levels – the main type of fat that accumulates in the liver. And the other benefits of eating fish regularly suggest that many of us would benefit from boosting our intake.

For example, in one study heart attacks were ten times less common among Greenland Inuits than in people from Denmark. On average, Greenland Inuits ate 14 g of omega-3 fatty acids a day, the Danes just 3 g.[3] Eating fish once or twice a week (or 30 g to 60 g a day) reduces the risk of dying from heart disease by 30–60 per cent.[5] Oily fish, the BDA points out, also keep your joints healthy, while omega-3 PUFAs are important for memory, intellectual performance and healthy vision. Your mother was right: fish really is brain food.

Omega-3 fatty acids – specifically docosahexaenoic acid (DHA) and eicosapentaenoic acid (EPA) – seem to be responsible for most of the health benefits of fish. We can make omega-3 fatty acids from another fat (alpha-linolenic acid) in green leafy vegetables, nuts, seeds and their oils. But it's a slow process. So, it's a good idea to boost levels by eating fish and seafood high in omega-3 fatty acids (Table 9.3).

The BDA advises that adults and children over 12 years of age should eat two portions of fish per week (a portion is about 140 g after cooking). One of these meals should be an oily fish. The BDA estimates that this will provide the equivalent of about 450 mg EPA/DHA per day. Omega-3 PUFA levels are higher in fresh fish. If you're eating canned fish, check the label to make sure processing has not depleted the omega-3 oils. It's also worth trying to check that the fish comes from sustainable stocks (<www.fishonline.org>).

If at first you don't like the taste, don't give up without trying some different fish and a few recipes. There are plenty of

Table 9.3 Examples of fish and seafood high in omega-3 fatty acids

Anchovy
Black cod (sablefish)
Crab
Dogfish (rock salmon)
Halibut
Herring
Mackerel
Mussels
Oysters
Pilchards
Rainbow trout
Sardines
Salmon
Tuna (especially bluefin)

Source: Adapted from the University of Michigan and the British Dietetic Association

suggestions on the Internet (e.g. <www.thefishsociety.co.uk>) and in cookbooks. For an island nation, our taste in fish is remarkably conservative. But if you really can't stomach the taste of oily fish you could try a supplement – provided you speak to your doctor first. If, for example, like many people with NAFLD you have diabetes, you may need to avoid omega-3 supplements, which might increase blood sugar levels. Finally, Andrew Weil points out that hemp oil and seeds (available from health shops and some larger supermarkets) also contain omega-3 fatty acids.

Vegetables, fruit and fibre

Our ancestors picked plants, fished and hunted. They ate vegetables, legumes, fruits and whole grains, which were usually fresh, often raw. This traditional diet – high in fibre and rich in vitamins and other micronutrients[6] – is a long way from processed foods loaded with sugar, salt, preservatives, colourings and flavourings. And a diet that's low in fruit and vegetables can contribute to liver disease. For example, as mentioned in Chapter 6, NASH patients also tend to have lower levels of certain carotenoids (yellow, orange and red pigments in plants). So, doctors and advocates of alternative detox tend to agree on at least one thing: cut down drastically on processed foods and increase your consumption of fruit and vegetables.

Boost your fibre intake

Dietary fibre (roughage) is the part of plants that humans cannot digest, such as the outer layers of sweetcorn, beans and wheat. There are two main types of fibre:

- Insoluble fibre remains largely intact as it moves through your digestive system. However, insoluble fibre makes defecation easier. Regular bowel movements may help remove toxins from the body and reduce the amount of toxins absorbed from foods.
- Soluble fibre dissolves in the water in the gut forming a gel, which soaks up fats. So, you absorb less fat from a meal, which brings your blood cholesterol levels down. Soluble fibre also releases sugar slowly, producing steadier blood levels after you eat. This can help stave off hunger pangs and so helps you lose weight, an issue we'll return to later in the chapter.

Dieticians recommend that healthy adults should eat at least 18 g of fibre a day. Currently, the average UK adult eats between 12 g and 14 g of fibre a day. So, you could boost your consumption of oats and oat bran; fruit and vegetables; nuts and seeds; pulses (such as peas, soya, lentils and chickpeas) and so on.

Whole grains

Whole grains are an especially good source of fibre. Grains – the seeds of cereals such as wheat, rye, barley, oats and rice – have three components:

1 Bran, the outer layer, is rich in fibre and packed with nutrients. Bran covers the germ and endosperm.
2 The germ develops into a new plant. So, the germ is packed with nutrients. Wheat germ, for example, contains high levels of vitamin E (page 55), folate (folic acid – page 45), zinc, magnesium and other vitamins and minerals.
3 The central area (endosperm) is largely starch, which provides the energy the germ needs to develop into a new plant.

Many food manufacturers refine grain by stripping off the bran and germ, and keeping the white endosperm. However, refining strips off most of the nutritional value. Indeed, whole grain contains up to 75 per cent more nutrients than refined cereals, the BDA points out. In addition to fibre, whole grains mop up tissue-damaging free radicals.

So, not surprisingly, a diet rich in whole grains helps you stay healthy. For example, the BDA notes that regularly eating whole-grain foods as part of a low-fat diet and a healthy lifestyle cuts the risk of heart disease by up to 30 per cent. Furthermore, in one study, men who ate, on average, 10.2 g of cereal fibre a day were 30 per cent less likely to develop type 2 diabetes than those who ate just 2.5 g a day. In another study, women who consumed an average of 7.5 g of cereal fibre a day were 28 per cent less likely to develop type 2 diabetes than women who ate 2 g a day.[2] As we've seen, type 2 diabetes is intimately linked to NAFLD (page 54).

Despite these benefits, 95 per cent of adults in the UK do not eat enough whole grains. Nearly a third do not eat any. The BDA advocates getting at least half your starchy carbohydrates from whole grains, which means two to three servings a day. Try eating more foods with 'whole' in front of the grain's name – such as whole-wheat pasta, wholegrain bread and whole oats.

Five portions of fruit and vegetables

Fruit and vegetables are rich in vitamins, minerals and fibre, which is why everyone – and not just people with chronic liver disease – should eat five portions of fruit and vegetables a day. A portion weighs about 80 g. The following list gives examples of the size of one portion:

- One medium-sized fruit (banana, apple, pear, orange)
- One slice of a large fruit (melon, pineapple, mango)
- Two smaller fruits (plums, satsumas, apricots, peaches)
- A dessert bowl full of salad
- Three heaped tablespoons of vegetables
- Three heaped tablespoons of pulses (chickpeas, lentils, beans)
- Two to three tablespoons (a handful) of grapes or berries
- One tablespoon of dried fruit
- One glass (150 ml) of unsweetened fruit or vegetable juice or smoothie. If you drink two or more glasses of juice a day, it still only counts as one portion.

Many detox diets emphasize the benefits of eating raw fruit and vegetables. Certainly, cooking can leach nutrients from fruits and vegetables. So, ideally, eat fruit and vegetables raw or cook using a small amount of unsalted water for the shortest time – you can also try lightly steaming and stir-frying. As mentioned before, try to avoid adding salt. And scrub rather than peel potatoes, carrots and so on: the skin is often a good source of nutrients.

Drinking smoothies is another great way to boost your intake of fruit and vegetables. However, some commercial smoothies contain extra sugar, honey, yoghurt or milk. So always check the label. Vegetable soups are a great way of boosting your intake of vegetables, but don't add salt and check the label of any you buy. It's often worth cooking extra quantities of soups and stews to freeze.

Seeds, nuts and legumes

Seeds, nuts and legumes are an excellent source of fibre and other nutrients. Plants use the energy stored in seeds to aid their early growth and development. So, seeds are relatively high in calories, which is worth bearing in mind if you are trying to shed a few pounds.

Not all the nuts we eat are, strictly, nuts. Brazil and cashew nuts are seeds, for example. Peanuts are legumes, more closely related to peas and lentils than chestnuts and hazelnuts. You can ponder such quibbles while eating a handful of almonds, cashews, walnuts, Brazils and pecans a day as snacks, sprinkled over your breakfast cereal and in baking.

Legumes are a cheap source of protein (page 87), are high in fibre and help control levels of fats in the blood. So, try to eat more of the following (continued overleaf):

- baked beans (although watch the sugar in some brands)
- kidney beans
- chickpeas (try a chickpea dahl, for example)
- red and green lentils
- mung beans
- butter beans
- black beans

The organic debate

Whether organic vegetables contain markedly higher levels of nutrients than conventionally farmed produce is scientifically contentious. One study evaluated 826 comparisons of the levels of micronutrients, such as vitamins and minerals, in organic and conventional foods from 33 studies. Just over half (56 per cent) of the studies found that micronutrient levels were higher in organic foods. On average, levels of micronutrients were approximately 6 per cent higher in organic vegetables and legumes compared with their conventionally grown counterparts.[7]

However, I believe that organically farmed products are, overall, healthier, not least because they avoid pesticides and chemical fertilizers. For example, pesticides seem to increase the risk of developing Parkinson's disease by 62 per cent among farmers and other exposed to high levels of these ubiquitous chemicals.[8] Whether the residues of modern pesticides and chemical fertilizers left on the food you buy in the high street (applied according to the UK's rigorous rules) cause widespread health problems is controversial. On the other hand, why eat them when you don't need to? And even a 6 per cent difference in nutrients could be worth having.

- split peas (pease pudding is one of my favourite foods – cheap and nutritious)
- haricot beans.

Vegetarian cook books are full of ideas to help you boost your bean consumption. You can also add beans to bulk up stews if you're cutting down on meat.

Another legume, the soya bean, is rich in polyunsaturated fats and low in saturated fat. The BDA notes that one portion of soya beans counts towards your recommended five portions of fruits and vegetables a day. Soya is also high in fibre and, unlike most other plant foods, contains all the essential amino acids (the building blocks of protein) you need to stay healthy. So, you could eat more soya products – including soya milk, tofu, tempeh and miso.

Eating to lose weight

As the bulging waistlines in any high street soon reveal, obesity is common. However, weight itself is not a very good guide to your risk of developing NAFLD, gall stones and other conditions linked to excess body fat, such as heart disease, hypertension, type 2 diabetes, breathing problems and some cancers. Weighting 14 stone is fine if you're 6 feet 5 inches. But you would be seriously obese if you were 5 feet 6 inches.

So, your body mass index (BMI) tells you whether you're overweight or obese based your height and weight. You should try to keep your BMI between 18.5 and 24.9 kg/m^2. Below this and you're dangerously underweight. A BMI between 25.0 and 29.9 kg/m^2 suggests that you are overweight. You're probably obese if your BMI exceeds 30.0 kg/m^2. For most people, BMI is a good guide to whether you're overweight. However, BMI may overestimate body fat in athletes, body builders and other muscular people (such as hod carriers). On the other hand, BMI may underestimate body fat in older persons and people who have lost muscle. (As we've seen, muscle wasting can be a symptom of chronic liver disease.)

Doctors and gyms can use a monitor to check your body fat. However, not all fat is equal. Abdominal obesity damages your health more than fat elsewhere in your body. So, waist size can tell you whether your health is at risk. The risk is especially marked in people of South Asian descent (Table 9.4).

Table 9.4 Waist sizes linked to an increased risk to your health

Group	Heath at risk	Health at high risk
Men	Over 94 cm (37 inches)	Over 102 cm (40 inches)
Women	Over 80 cm (32 inches)	Over 88 cm (35 inches)
South Asian men		Over 90 cm (36 inches)
South Asian women		Over 80 cm (32 inches)

Source: Adapted from the British Heart Foundation

So, many of us need to shed a few pounds. Unfortunately, losing weight is not easy – whatever the latest fad diets would have you believe. After all, millions of years of evolution drive us to consume food in times of feast to help us survive times of famine. And you can't stop eating as you can quit smoking or drinking excessive amounts of alcohol.

Indeed, crash dieting can be counterproductive and may even increase the risk of some liver diseases. For example, crash diets can

Tips to help you lose weight

- Keep a food diary and record everything that you eat and drink for a couple of weeks. This helps you see where you inadvertently pile on the extra calories: the odd biscuit here, the extra glass of wine or full-fat latte there. It all adds up. A food diary can also help you see if you're eating fatty or high-salt food without realizing.
- Set specific goals. Don't say that you want to lose weight; rather, resolve to lose 2 stone by Christmas.
- Think about how you tried to lose weight in the past. What techniques and diets worked? Which failed to make a difference? Which were you unable to stick to? Did a support group help?
- Don't let a slip-up derail your diet. Try to identify why you indulged – what were the triggers? A particular occasion? Do you comfort eat? Once you know why you slipped you can develop strategies to stop future slip-ups.
- Begin your diet when you're at home over a weekend or a holiday and you don't have a celebration (such as Christmas or a birthday) planned. It's tougher changing your diet on a Monday morning or when you're away on business in a hotel faced with fat-packed food, caffeine-rich drinks and calorie-laden alcohol.

cause the liver to release more cholesterol into bile, increasing your risk of gall stones (page 77). Crash dieting also means that the gall bladder does not empty properly, which makes gall stones even more likely. So, set yourself a realistic target weight (using the BMI) and a reasonable time. Eating between 500 and 1000 calories less each day can reduce body weight (assuming your BMI is stable) by between 0.5 and 1.0 kg each week.[6] Steadily losing around a pound or two a week reduces your chances of putting it back on again. But remember, you'll lose weight more quickly in the first few weeks as you burn off the glycogen stores (page 7) in your liver before you start to lose fat.

If all this fails, try talking to your GP or pharmacist. (Make sure they know you have chronic liver disease and any other ailments.) A growing number of medicines may help kick-start your weight loss. None offers a magic cure for being overweight. You'll still need to change your lifestyle. However, they may help put you on the right course towards weight loss.

Boost your exercise

You can lose weight by reducing the amount of calories you consume and you can lose weight by increasing the amount you burn off. And of course you'll lose weight quicker if you do both. Ideally, you should be moderately active for at least 30 minutes on at least 5 days – and ideally every day – a week. It does not all have to be in one go. You can exercise for 15 minutes twice a day, for example.

You should aim to exercise until you are breathing harder than usual, but not so hard that you can't hold a conversation. You should feel that your heart is beating faster than usual and you've begun to sweat. However, if you experience chest pain, or feel faint or otherwise unwell stop exercising and see your doctor.

You should aim to integrate exercise into your everyday life. If you've been exercising regularly for a year, you'll lose about half your cardiovascular fitness in just 3 months if you stop. So, find a type of exercise that suits you and that fits into your lifestyle. If you're someone who doesn't like exercise classes and you join a gym some distance from home or work, you're less likely to stick to the programme. That's one of the reasons that walking is such good exercise. The American Heart Association suggests taking at least 10,000 steps a day. You could use a pedometer to ensure you walk far enough.

Tips for being more active

There are plenty of opportunities to become more active as you go about your day-to-day life, such as:

- Walk to the local shops instead of taking the car.
- Ride a bike to work instead of travelling by car or public transport.
- Park a 15-minute walk from your place of work.
- If you take the bus, tube or metro, get off one or two stops early.
- Use the stairs instead of the lift.
- Clean the house regularly and wash your car by hand.
- Grow your own vegetables – a great way to boost consumption, they also taste better.
- Look for country parks and nature reserves in your area. There are more than 400 country parks in England alone. The Natural England and the Royal Society for the Protection of Birds websites are good places to start: (<www.naturalengland.org.uk/ourwork/enjoying/places/countryparks/countryparksnetwork/findacountrypark> and <www.rspb.org.uk/reserves>).

Diet and detox

Eating a healthy, balanced diet is the foundation of most detox regimens. Some detox diets suggest eating fruit and vegetables exclusively (and often raw) for anything between a day and a week. Almost all complementary therapists recommend that you eat nutrient-rich foods, lean meat or a vegetarian diet and eliminate sugar, white flour, additives and so on. Few doctors would disagree.

You also need to drink plenty of water and herbal teas. Complementary therapists claim this helps flush toxins out of your body. Certainly, scientific studies show that even mild dehydration can cause a variety of symptoms including: reduced vigilance and concentration; poor memory; increased tension or anxiety; fatigue and headache.[9, 10, 11]

Headaches are among the most common symptoms that complementary practitioners link to toxic overload. Whether or not this is true, increasing the amount of water you drink may help limit headaches' impact on your day-to-day life. For example, one study included 102 people who experienced at least two moderately intense headaches (such as tension headaches and migraine) or at least five mildly intense headaches per month and drank less than 2.5 litres of fluid daily. The researchers asked 52 of these people to increase the amount of water they drank by 1.5 litres a day.[11]

After 3 months, people who increased the amount of water they drank reported an improved quality of life compared with those who did not increase their water consumption (called controls). And almost half (47 per cent) of those who increased water consumption reported 'much improvement' (at least 6 points on a 10-point scale) in their headaches compared with 25 per cent of controls. Drinking more water did not change the number of days that subjects experienced at least moderate headaches. So, it's worth boosting the amount of water you drink if you have regular headaches.[11]

In general, the NHS notes that adults should drink 1.2 litres (6–8 glasses of water) each day. Remember that alcohol abuse and diabetes can leave you dehydrated. If you feel thirsty for long periods, you're not drinking enough. And increase your intake during exercise or hot weather, if you feel lightheaded, pass dark-coloured urine or haven't passed urine within 6 hours. If you regularly feel thirsty, despite maintaining your fluid intake, you should see your doctor. Excessive thirst can be a sign of diabetes (page 58).

Nevertheless, as we'll see in the Chapter 10, many doctors remain sceptical about the benefits of other aspects of detox. So, whether or not the claims for detox are true, eating a healthy diet is certainly good for your health – and you'll feel better.

10

Using herbs to cleanse the liver

Humanity has long sought treatments for liver diseases. According to Ronald Hutton's *The Stations of the Sun*, an eleventh century Anglo-Saxon medical book suggested that vervain (*Verbena*) gathered on Midsummer's Day alleviated liver problems. David Conway comments that traditional British herbalists used several other herbal liver tonics, including agrimony (once called liverwort), centaury, dandelion, rosemary and sage.

Other medical traditions worldwide also used herbs to bolster hepatic health. Lise Manniche points out that the ancient Egyptians treated liver problems with chicory (*Cichorium intybus*) mixed with wine. Healers in Pharaonic Egypt advocated a mixture of white lotus, ziziphus, juniper berries, frankincense, wine and small beer for jaundice, while the Assyrians suggested white mustard (*Sinapis alba*) for the same condition. Traditional Islamic healers used sweet flag (*Acorus calamus*) to alleviate liver inflammation, Manniche adds. And radish juice (*Raphanus sativus*) is a traditional treatment for gall stones.

More recently, the conventional (allopathic) treatments we've mentioned over the course of the book have transformed management of liver disease. Nevertheless, people with chronic liver disease often try alternative and complementary treatments, some of which we'll also consider in Chapter 11. Many other people try to detox to prevent liver disease and enhance their well-being and vitality.

Certainly, a growing number of scientific studies suggest that some herbs protect the liver, milk thistle probably being the most famous. Ironically, however, some herbal remedies are potent hepatic poisons. So, in this chapter, we'll look at some herbs that may help people with liver disease and how you can use them safely. In all cases, you should use these approaches to bolster a healthy lifestyle and complement, rather than replace, any conventional treatments your doctor suggests.

Detoxification and 'cleanses'

As we saw in Chapter 9, a healthy balanced diet can protect your liver, which means you're better able to cope with toxins in the environment, in your food and produced as by-products by your body. However, some people go further, using a variety of 'treatments': from herbal concoctions, to enemas, to extreme diets and fasting, to 'detox'. So, some alternative practitioners use liver flushes and cleanses to, they claim, drive harmful chemicals and metabolic by-products from the body – it's easy to find examples on the Internet. And, as we've seen, the liver controls the levels of certain hormones. This means, the practitioners claim, that flushes can help tackle hormonal imbalances.

However, critics note that very little evidence from scientific studies supports these approaches.[1] For example, the American Cancer Society notes that the current evidence 'does not support claims that liver flushes are useful for preventing or treating cancer or any other diseases'. And, occasionally, detox does more harm than good – as we'll see.

Part of the problem is that 'toxin' is, scientifically speaking, rather vague. The term traces its origins to *toxicon,* the ancient Greek word for bow poison. In turn, *toxicon* may derive from the poison that the Scythians smeared on their arrows.[2] For many alternative and complementary practitioners, toxins are modern poisoned arrows let slip by alcohol, cigarettes, diet, pollution, pesticides, heavy metals and so on.

According to advocates of detox, if our liver or gastrointestinal tract performs poorly, levels of toxins in our body rise. This toxic overload, some complementary practitioners claim, can cause a range of symptoms including poor complexion, lethargy, mental slowness, gastrointestinal upsets, muscular aches and pains, and headaches. Detox uses diets, herbs, vitamins, colonic irrigation and enemas, saunas, homeopathic remedies and a variety of other interventions to remove the toxins.[1]

A liver flush, for example, might involving drinking a range of juices, Epsom salts and oils, along with certain herbs or preparations of enzymes. You'll flush for a couple days and pass several bowel movements. However, the composition of the flush may vary between practitioners and the various formulations bought on the Internet. (I would advise against buying any product – conventional medicine, supplement or alternative formulation – over the Internet unless you are *absolutely* sure the site is reputable.)

Some people experience nausea, vomiting and diarrhoea during the flush and an oily preparation can trigger contraction of the gallbladder and any stones could lodge in the duct, The American Cancer Society warns. And as we'll see, some herbs can damage the liver. So, you need to be careful about any flush, the practitioner suggesting the cleanse and the components of the formulation. Check carefully before you flush.

On the other hand, scientific studies suggest that air pollution (a cocktail of toxic chemicals) increases the risk of death from conditions of the heart and blood vessels (cardiovascular disease).[3] A study that integrated the results from 34 previous investigations estimated that, depending on the chemical, air pollution accounts for between around 1 in 160 (0.6 per cent) and 1 in 22 (4.5 per cent) heart attacks.[3]

Furthermore, nitrogen dioxide produced by road vehicles, power plants, some factories and so on seems to exacerbate asthma symptoms and undermines how well your lungs work. The effect is especially marked in young children and elderly people.[4] As we noted when we looked at organic food, exposure to relatively high levels of pesticide, either at work or other circumstances such as gardening, seems to cause some cases of Parkinson's disease.[5]

The health risks of excessive levels of heavy metals such as lead, mercury and copper (see Wilson's disease – page 73) are beyond debate. Mercury poisoning can undermine hand–eye coordination, and causes heart, hormonal and immune problems.[6] Indeed, in humans, mercury accumulates in the liver, kidney and spleen.[7] So, the link between ill-health and toxins does not seem that unlikely.

Nevertheless, critics counter that little scientific evidence supports the detox approaches suggested by complementary practitioners. And, they add, some detox approaches carry risks. Not eating a healthy diet or prolonged fasting can lead to nutritional deficiencies, for example. As we'll see, some herbs can cause liver toxicity, while colonic irrigation can perforate the bowel.[1]

Vitamins and minerals

As mentioned in Chapter 1, the liver stores vitamin A. In the early days of Arctic exploration, some adventurers died after eating the livers of polar bears, which contain very high levels of vitamin A. And some people have developed hepatotoxicity after taking high doses (so-called mega-doses) of vitamin A. Most people who developed toxicity regularly consumed more than 50,000 IU of vitamin A daily. However, levels of liver enzymes can rise after taking approximately 25,000 IU per day and in rare cases people regularly taking this dose of vitamin A can develop severe hepatotoxicity.[8]

Large doses (100–125 mg/day) of vanadium improve cells' sensitivity to insulin in humans, which, in theory at least, may help NAFLD (page 58). But at these doses, vanadium tends to cause side effects, such as abdominal discomfort, diarrhoea, nausea, gas, loss of energy and even a green tongue.[9] Most multivitamin and mineral preparations contain levels well within safe daily limits,[10] even for people with liver disease. But it's sensible to be cautious: avoid very high doses and, if you have any disease, check with your doctor before taking any supplement.

Furthermore, some alternative healers believe that detox drives out the toxins that have accumulated (often, they say, over years) in the liver and other tissues. They suggest that this toxic 'tsunami' can produce a detox 'crisis', characterized by unpleasant symptoms including headaches, fatigue and abdominal discomfort. In some cases, the healer and the person undergoing detox can mistake adverse events for a crisis. So, you need to be careful if you experience any unexpected symptoms during detox.

Nevertheless, some people undoubtedly feel better after detox, especially if it's relatively gentle. So, if you want to try, check with your doctor first, especially if you have liver disease or any other medical condition. Then ensure that you consult a registered practitioner, such as one recognized by the General Regulatory Council for Complementary Therapies. Read up on the approach you're planning to use and make sure you understand the risks and benefits.

Herbal treatments

In 1960, archaeologists discovered a Neanderthal skeleton buried in caves in Shanidar, northern Iraq. Several plants still used by modern herbalists, including cornflower, groundsel and yarrow, surrounded the 40,000-year-old remains.

Almost certainly, the plants were not there by accident and probably formed part of the Neanderthals' pharmacy. Indeed, the herbs represent the two faces of herbal treatments for liver disease. Yarrow (*Achillea millefolium*) is a traditional treatment for liver and gall bladder disease.[11] Common groundsel (*Senecio vulgaris*), although used in some traditional herbal remedies, can cause liver damage.[12]

Today, herbs are the main source of medicines for much of humanity. And they remain popular in countries able to afford modern medicine. Indeed, many medicines prescribed by your doctor and pharmacist – even for serious diseases – trace their origins to herbs. For instance:

- In 1763, the English chaplain Edward Stone found that willow bark alleviated ague, a fever linked to malaria, which was rife in England at the time. Aspirin is a chemically modified, less toxic version of the active ingredient in willow bark.
- Metformin (page 58), one of the most important diabetes drugs, is a chemical modification of a substance in the French lilac (*Galega officinalis*). Medieval healers used French lilac to relieve urinary problems. (Diabetic patients produce large volumes of urine.)
- In 1962, a botanist named Arthur Barclay peeled some bark from a Pacific Yew tree (*Taxus brevifolia*) growing in the Gifford Pinchot National Forest in north-eastern USA. Today, oncologists use a drug called paclitaxel, extracted from yew bark, to treat various malignancies including lung, breast and ovarian cancer.[13]

In other words, plant-derived drugs are potentially potent medicines. So everyone taking a medicine for any disease *must* speak to a doctor before taking a herbal treatment, even if you can buy it from a health shop.

Herbal detox

Against this background, a growing body of scientific evidence suggests that certain herbs alleviate liver diseases and bolster hepatic health. For example, Indian Ayurvedic medicine, which is among the world's richest and longest-established healing traditions, stresses the importance of diet and herbal remedies to maintain well-being. Ayurvedic healers use around 1,200 plants to treat a wide range of illnesses, including 90 herbs in some 300 preparations for jaundice and chronic liver disease alone. Researchers have not scientifically investigated all of these, but some seem to alleviate liver problems.[14]

For instance, the arjun tree (*Terminalia arjuna*) grows on river banks in Bengal as well as in south and central India. Indian healers traditionally used the arjun tree as a heart tonic. In experiments using mice, extracts of the tree's smooth grey bark seem to protect the liver from damage by carbon tetrachloride, one of the most potent hepatic toxins.[15]

Why traditional herbs for the liver may work

Herbs could help bolster hepatic health in several ways including:[14]

- Some herbs improve gastrointestinal function. For example, alleviating constipation can reduce the absorption of substances that could damage the liver.
- Several herbs seem to protect liver cells by reducing inflammation and improving blood flow.
- Chemicals in certain herbs may inhibit the liver enzymes that convert drugs to toxic metabolites (page 5).
- Viruses can affect plants as well as humans. So plants have evolved antiviral chemicals, many of which coincidentally attack human viruses, including some of those responsible for hepatitis. For example, astragalus (*Astragalus membranaceus*), which is widely used in traditional Chinese medicine to, among other roles, fight infections, counter fatigue and strengthen the lungs, inhibits HBV replication in experimental animals. As the effect is relatively weak, astragalus is only suitable as a supplement to conventional medicines.[16]
- Certain herbs seem to bolster protein production and reduce hepatic fibrosis and scarring, which aids liver regeneration.

Another herb, called katuka (*Picrorhiza kurroa* Royle ex Benth), grows in the Himalayas. Katuka, which traditional Indian healers use to treat jaundice, also seems to protect the liver against damage from carbon tetrachloride, paracetamol and some other toxins. Furthermore, a widely used traditional Ayurvedic treatment that contains katuka treats viral hepatitis. In animal experiments, katuka seems to reverse the fatty changes characteristic of NAFLD.[17] As always, it's best to be treated by an experienced qualified healer: contact the Ayurvedic Practitioners Association or the British Association of Accredited Ayurvedic Practitioners.

Milk thistle

Closer to home, milk thistle (*Silybum marianum*), a member of the same botanical family as daisies and sunflowers, grows wild across southern Europe, southern Russia, Asia Minor and North Africa.[18] Since antiquity, European healers have used milk thistle to treat liver and gall bladder disorders, including hepatitis, cirrhosis and jaundice, as well as protecting against chemical poisons, snakebites, insect stings, mushroom poisoning and alcohol.[18]

For instance, the Greek physician Pedanius Dioscorides collected local herbs as he travelled around the Roman Empire with Nero's army. Around AD 70, Dioscorides published *De Materia Medica* (one of the first herbals) and described using tea made from milk thistle to treat the bite of serpents. (Several snake venoms can damage the liver – after all, the liver helps remove toxins from our blood.)

The milk thistle legend

According to legend, Mary once nursed Jesus in a bower made from milk thistle. A drop of the Virgin Mary's milk fell on the plant, producing the white veins that run through the plant's shiny, spiky, scalloped-edged leaves. The legend inspired some of the plant's other names, which include Marian thistle; Mary thistle; St Mary's thistle; Our Lady's thistle; Blessed Virgin thistle; and Holy thistle. Folk traditions say that nursing mothers would benefit from the milk thistle. Scientific studies have confirmed that the active ingredients may increase breast milk production,[18] although you should *never* take any herb or medicine while breastfeeding until you have checked with your doctor.

Around the same time, the Roman writer Pliny the Elder (AD 23–79) said that a mix of milk thistle and honey 'carried off bile'. The plant is also part of traditional Indian and Chinese medicines. Once again, scientific studies suggest that these herbal traditions contain more than a grain of truth.[18]

Scientists now know that milk thistle contains several active chemicals. The extract of milk thistle used commonly, called silymarin, contains four chemicals. One of these – silibinin (silybin) – accounts for about 50 to 70 per cent of silymarin. Experimental studies suggest that silibinin alone and silymarin:

- protect the liver from toxins;
- mop up tissue-damaging free radicals;
- counter inflammation;
- reduce fibrosis (page 12);
- increase protein production, which helps repair damaged hepatocytes;
- reduce the amount of some poisons (including certain toxins from mushrooms) absorbed by liver cells. As mentioned above, protecting against mushroom poisoning is one of milk thistle's traditional roles;[18]
- may directly kill cancer cells, which boosts the effectiveness of conventional chemotherapies.[18]

Does milk thistle work in humans?

Several studies suggest that milk thistle, silymarin and silibinin alleviate liver diseases, including cirrhosis and hepatitis. However, drawing definitive conclusions about milk thistle's benefits is difficult. The studies assessed various preparations and doses. Treatment duration ranged from a few days to many years. And the patients included differed from study to study. For example, people in studies of alcohol-related liver disease varied in the amount they previously drank, whether they were abstinent or not during treatment with milk thistle, and the severity of liver damage.[18]

Despite these differences, silymarin seems to effectively treat poisoning with the aptly named death cap mushroom (*Amanita phalloides*) and may alleviate alcohol-induced liver diseases, especially Child–Pugh class A cirrhosis (page 26). In alcoholic liver disease, silymarin seems to decrease abnormal levels of certain liver enzymes (including ALT and AST – page 25), normalize damaged areas of the liver and reduce the telltale changes that herald the progression of fibrosis.[18]

Silymarin does not inhibit replication of viruses responsible for hepatitis (Chapter 4). Nevertheless, milk thistle seems to reduce the severity of the inflammation triggered by hepatitis viruses, which contributes to the liver damage and symptoms.[18] However, one study found that high doses of silymarin did not reduce levels of the liver enzyme ALT (page 25) in people with chronic HCV who did not respond to interferon.[19] On the other hand, these patients are, obviously, very difficult to treat – after all they did not respond to some of the most powerful antivirals in the allopathic armoury. So perhaps the lack of success is not that surprising.

Milk thistle rarely causes side effects at the usual dose of 140–400 mg a day. Indeed, no one of a group of patients with one of several liver disorders developed side effects after receiving silymarin (600–800 mg daily) for 6 months. Overall, around 1 in 100 people who took silymarin (560 mg a day) for 8 weeks developed side effects, which included short-lived gastrointestinal problems, such as bloating, nausea, dyspepsia and diarrhoea. At very high doses (more than 1500 mg a day), silymarin may be a laxative.[18] Nevertheless, speak to your doctor before using any herbal treatment for liver disease or another condition, and stop taking the supplement if you feel unwell.

Milk thistle as a mental tonic

David Conway remarks that European herbalists used milk thistle as an antidepressant and as a heart, kidney and brain tonic. Indeed, some herbalists believe that milk thistle helps tackle memory loss caused by old age or sickness. As we've seen, liver disease can cause depression and other mental symptoms. Perhaps part of the milk thistle's reputation as an antidepressant and mental tonic arises because the herb counters liver problems and, as a result, improves hepatic encephalopathy (page 16). However, this is speculation on my part. As an aside, Jennifer Harper remarks that traditional Chinese healers regard depression and melancholy as the consequence of 'liver stagnation'.

Liquorice

Many people now think of liquorice as long 'laces', Catherine wheels, 'allsorts' and other sweets. However, liquorice, which belongs to a group of plants called *Glycyrrhiza*, meaning sweet root, has a longer history and more diverse uses than most people realize. Indeed, our ancestors used liquorice even before the rise of the ancient Babylonian and Egyptian civilizations, both of which valued the plant highly. The ancient Greeks used liquorice to treat asthma and dry cough and to prevent thirst. In Chinese medicine, liquorice root (called *gan cao*) is one of the longest established and most widely used herbs for diseases as diverse as tuberculosis and stomach ulcers.[20]

A chemical called glycyrrhizin seems to be responsible for many of liquorice's benefits. Glycyrrhizin reduces inflammation, mops up free radicals (page 56), modulates the immune system[21] and seems to protect the liver from paracetamol, carbon tetrachloride and other toxins. Furthermore, liquorice seems to attack several parasites, bacteria and viruses, including hepatitis A, B and C.[22]

For example, one study examined liquorice in 66 people with NAFLD. All showed raised levels of liver enzymes (page 24) before treatment. Half the group received 2 g of an extract of liquorice root a day for 2 months. The remainder received an inactive placebo. Liquorice normalized levels of ALT and AST,[21] suggesting that the plant may help reverse damage caused by NAFLD. While further studies are needed to fully characterize the benefits, liquorice seems to offer a valuable liver 'tonic'.

Garlic

As David Conway noted, garlic 'is something of a herbal panacea', used by traditional herbalists to treat rheumatism and lung disease, and bolster resistance to infection. Holding a slice between a sore tooth and the gum can relieve toothache – a trick I've used on occasion.

And a growing body of evidence suggests that garlic may help liver diseases. For example, in experiments using rats, S-allylmercaptocysteine (a chemical in garlic) reduced NAFLD-induced liver injury, fat accumulation, collagen production (an early step in fibrosis) and levels of free fatty acids (page 7).[23] In rats, raw garlic reduced the accumulation of some heavy metals (including cadmium and mercury) in the liver.[24] There is even experimental evidence that garlic extracts can reverse fibrosis, regenerate liver tissue and restore hepatic function.[25] Human studies now need to confirm these promising results.

So, use garlic liberally in your cooking. Garlic's really easy to grow, even in pots on the patio. Buy an organic bulb, ideally from the UK, and gently separate the cloves. (You can also buy cloves to plant from garden centres.) Discard any cloves that feel slightly soft. Then plant the cloves pointed end up. My home-grown garlic certainly tastes more potent than that bought from the supermarket.

Using herbs safely

While many herbs improve liver function and seem to protect against hepatic poisons, some can trigger side effects. Liquorice, for example, can cause several adverse events, especially at high doses, including dangerous increases in blood pressure, abnormal changes in heart rhythm, headache, short-lived visual loss, and muscle weakness.[21,22] And some herbal remedies seem to cause liver damage (Table 10.1).

Kava kava and liver disease

The kava kava (*Piper methysticum*) shrub from some islands in the South Pacific illustrates the risk of liver damage associated with certain herbs. Drinking a traditional beverage – kava derives its name from the Polynesian word *awa* meaning bitter – made from the herb produces mild intoxication, and is central to many cere-monial and social gatherings in Pacific Island societies. In addition, traditional healers used kava to treat numerous diseases including gonorrhoea, syphilis, cystitis and insomnia. In Europe, herbalists used kava to treat anxiety. Clinical trials have suggested that kava works.[26]

However, heavy consumption of kava – up to 100 times the recommended medical dose – over a long time can cause a range of problems, including malnutrition, weight loss, a rash, kidney disease and liver problems. Even at recommended therapeutic doses, kava can cause mild, short-lived adverse effects such as redness of the skin, headache and liver damage.[26] Indeed, by 2006

Table 10.1 Some herbal remedies linked to liver damage[10,26]

Common name	Latin name	Comments
Amanita mushrooms	Species of *Amanita*, such as *A. muscaria*	Known as fly agaric
Asafetida	*Ferula assafoetida*	An Indian herb also called giant fennel and *Jowani badian*
Chaparral	*Larrea tridentata*	A native American herb
Comfrey	Species of *Symphytum*, such as *S. officinale*	Traditionally used to help bones heal
Echinacea	Species of *Echinacea*	Sometimes used to boost the immune system and help fight colds
Gentian	Species of *Gentiana*	Used in some soft and alcoholic drinks
Germander	Species of *Teucrium*	Traditionally used for gout and as a tonic
Jin bu huan	*Lycopodium serratum*	A traditional Chinese herbal sedative and analgesic
Kava kava	*Piper methysticum*	See discussion in this chapter
Mistletoe	*Viscum album* and related species	Apart from the traditional use at Christmas, doctors in some European countries prescribe mistletoe extracts as a cancer treatment
Pennyroyal	*Mentha pulegium*	Traditionally used for menstrual problems, abortions, upset stomach
Senna	*Senna alexandrina* (sometimes called Cassia officinalis)	Fruit extracts widely used as laxatives
Valerian	*Valeriana officinalis*	Used in some 'natural' remedies for sleep disorders; check the label

the Food Standards Agency had received 110 reports over several years of people who had experienced severe liver damage that was possibly caused by kava kava. Of these, 11 patients suffered irreversible liver failure and received a liver transplant. Nine people died.

However, it's worth noting, that in 2006 *alone,* paracetamol, which remains on sale, contributed to 309 deaths (page 81).

Herbal interactions

Some herbs can interfere with conventional medicines. As we saw in Chapter 1, the liver produces enzymes that break down medicines. If another chemical blocks these metabolic enzymes, the resulting increase in blood level of the medicine can cause side effects.

If a herbal treatment induces the metabolic enzyme that breaks down another drug, the resulting decrease in blood levels of the medicine can undermine its effectiveness. For example, St John's wort (*Hypericum perforatum*) is as effective at alleviating mild depression as the usual doses of conventional antidepressants – and is less likely to cause side effects. Nevertheless, St John's wort induces several cytochrome P450 enzymes (page 5) and, as a result, undermines the effectiveness of a wide range of drugs including:

- digoxin, used for heart failure and abnormal heart rhythms;
- indinavir, a treatment for HIV;
- amitriptyline, another antidepressant;
- ciclosporin (cyclosporin), used to prevent people from rejecting transplanted organs;
- warfarin, which prevents dangerous blood clots;
- oral contraceptives.[26]

The risk of interactions is one reason why it's so important to tell your pharmacist, GP or nurse that you are also taking a herbal medicine. You should also tell your medical herbalist about any conventional drugs you're taking.

A complicated mix

Pharmacologists (scientists who research drugs) tend to study a single, specific chemical extracted from the herb – as we've seen in the studies of milk thistle and garlic. However, plants contain a mixture of chemicals, several of which can contribute to the herb's benefits. In *Health and Healing*, Andrew Weil notes, for example, that opium contains 22 active ingredients. To complicate matters further, many herbal formulations contain several different plants: some traditional Chinese medicines contain more than 20 components, for instance. As the herbs may influence each other, assessing the risk of side effects and interactions with conventional medicines can prove difficult.

And remember that the amount of active drug in an herb is less than the amount in a conventional medicine. While this means that you are less likely to experience side effects, it also means that the benefits can take longer to emerge or the improvement may not be as marked. Nevertheless, if you feel that you are not benefiting after 3 months or so, or you develop any changes that could be side effects, stop taking the formulation and see your medical herbalist.

Unfortunately, few complementary therapies undergo the same rigorous testing as modern medicines. But clinical studies are expensive and pharmaceutical companies fund most trials. So, this lack of studies is not that surprising. It's worth remembering that no evidence of effectiveness is not necessarily the same as evidence of no effect. Nevertheless, as mentioned above, if you fail to see any benefits after 3 months you should stop using the herb. And before you embark on a course of herbal supplements, speak to your doctor. Not all products include the detailed information you need to take the supplement safely.

So, if you decide to try herbal remedies or other supplements make sure you buy reputable preparations from a shop with knowledgeable staff. You should also look for standardized extracts: the amount of active ingredient can vary depending where it is grown and when it is harvested. (That may be why some traditional herbals suggest gathering the plant at a particular time or associate the herb with a particular astrological sign.) Rather than treating yourself using herbs, it's best to consult a qualified medical herbalist and make sure they know you have liver disease or any other medical condition. Nevertheless, used appropriately, herbs can help you cleanse and protect your liver.

11

Living with liver disease

As we've seen, liver diseases typically develop slowly over many years. This offers you a window of opportunity to reduce the risk that the disease will progress by, for example, cutting down on your alcohol consumption, eating a healthy diet and taking the treatments prescribed by your doctor. In this chapter, we'll look at some other ways that may help you live with liver disease.

Quit smoking

Nicotine, the addictive chemical in tobacco, and the plant's scientific name (*Nicotiana tabacum*) 'honour' Jean Nicot de Villemain (1530–1600), the French ambassador to Portugal who introduced tobacco to Parisian society when he returned from Lisbon in 1561. Tobacco rapidly became fashionable. However, more than 400 years later, smoking is increasingly socially unacceptable – just look at the huddles of smokers outside offices, pubs and restaurants.

Indeed, the proportion of the UK population who smoke is declining. During the 1940s around 70 per cent of men and 40 per cent of women smoked. According to government statistics, in 2009 22 per cent of men and 20 per cent of women in England smoked. That's a welcome fall. But about 8.8 million smokers still put their lives at risk. For example:

- Around half of those who do not quit smoking die prematurely from their addiction.
- Smokers are roughly twice as likely to die from cancer as non-smokers are.
- Smoking increases the likelihood of suffering a stroke up to threefold.
- Smoking underlies one-fifth of deaths among middle-aged people.
- Smoking causes around half of all cases of heart disease.

On the other hand, quitting reduces your likelihood of developing most smoking-related diseases. According to the Department of Health:

- A lifelong smoker dies, on average, around 10 years sooner than they otherwise would.
- A person who stops smoking at 30 or 40 years of age gains, on average, 10 and 9 years of life, respectively.
- Even a 60-year-old gains 3 years of life by quitting.

The dangers to your family

If the benefits to your health are not enough to make you quit, think of the harm you're doing to your loved ones. Second-hand smoke contains more than 4,000 chemicals, including about 50 carcinogens. This cocktail of chemical toxins increases the risk of serious diseases – including cancer, heart disease, asthma and sudden infant death syndrome – in people who inhale second-hand smoke. For example, the risks that a woman who has never smoked will develop lung cancer or heart disease are 24 and 30 per cent greater, respectively, if she lives with a smoker.

Making quitting easier

Fewer than 1 in every 30 smokers manages to quit each year, and more than half of these relapse within a year. And ideally you need to quit, not cut down. People who reduce the number of cigarettes they smoke usually inhale more deeply to get the same amount of nicotine. Nevertheless, cutting back seems to increase the likelihood that you'll eventually quit by, in some studies, 70 per cent compared with those who never cut back. In other words, reduction can take you a large step towards kicking the habit. But don't stop there.

You'll need to deal with nicotine's withdrawal symptoms, which can leave you irritable, restless and anxious, experiencing insomnia and suffering intense cravings for a cigarette. In general, withdrawal symptoms abate over 2 weeks or so. However, nicotine replacement therapy (NRT) can help you cope with the withdrawal symptoms. You can chose from various types of NRT. Patches reduce withdrawal symptoms, but have a relatively slow onset of action.

Table 11.1 Likelihood of smoking cessation 12 months after quitting[1]

	Compared with control*	Compared with varenicline
Combinations of different nicotine replacement therapies	34 per cent more effective	Varenicline 78 per cent more effective
Standard-dose (less than 22 mg) nicotine patches	48 per cent more effective	Varenicline 65 per cent more effective
High-dose nicotine patches	69 per cent more effective	Varenicline 47 per cent more effective
Bupropion	40 per cent more effective	Varenicline 61 per cent more effective
Varenicline	139 per cent more effective	–

*One group received the treatment to aid cessation; the 'control' group did not – they may have received an inert placebo.

Nicotine chewing gum, lozenges, inhalers and nasal spray act more quickly. Talk to your pharmacist or GP to find the right combination for use.

If you still find quitting tough even after trying NRT, doctors can prescribe other treatments, such as bupropion and varenicline. Indeed, varenicline seems to be the most effective smoking cessation aid based on the result of 146 studies (Table 11.1).[1] But there is no quick fix. You'll still need to be committed to quitting.

Tips to help you quit

Breaking tobacco's hold is tough. After all, on some measures, nicotine is more addictive than heroin or cocaine. But, in addition to using NRT, a few hints may make life easier:

- Set a quit date when you will stop completely. Plan ahead· keep a diary of problems and situations that tempt you to light up, such as stress, coffee, meals, pubs or work breaks. Then try to find alternatives.
- Try to find something to take your mind off smoking. If you find yourself smoking when you get home in the evening, try a

new hobby or exercise. If you find car journeys boring without a cigarette, listen to an audio book or a comedy CD. Most people find that the craving for a cigarette usually only lasts a couple of minutes.

- Smoking is expensive. Keep a note of how much you save, and spend at least some of it on something for yourself.
- Tackle stress. You could try relaxation therapies.
- Get a free quit smoking pack from the NHS Smoking Helpline (0800 022 4 332).
- Ask if your area offers NHS antismoking clinics, often at a doctor's surgery. These clinics offer advice, support and, when appropriate, a supply of NRT.
- Think about hypnotherapy. If you would like to try this, ask your doctor for a recommendation or contact the British Association of Medical Hypnosis.

You may also need to deal with hunger pangs. Military commanders from the Thirty Years War to World War I encouraged smoking to blunt fear and hunger. But try to avoid reaching for the sweet packet, which may mean you put on weight. In one study, people who quit smoking gained 1.12 kg during the month after quitting and 4.67 kg after a year.[2] Watching the consumption of sweet items and junk foods can help you control your weight. However, it's worth noting that 16 per cent of people lost weight after quitting, 37 per cent gained less than 5 kg, and 13 per cent gained more than 10 kg.[2] Try the weight loss tips on page 95. If you really crave sugar, try some sweet-tasting foods instead, such as dates, kiwi fruit and pineapple.

Keep trying

Nicotine is incredibly addictive and, not surprisingly, many people do not manage to quit the first time they try. But if you relapse, try not to become too dispirited. Regard it as a temporary setback, set another quit date and try again.

It's also worth trying to identify why you relapsed. Were you stressed out? If so, why? Was smoking linked to a particular time, place or event? Once you know why you slipped you can develop strategies to stop the problem in the future.

The emotional turmoil

Liver disease can be distressing, debilitating and even disabling. If you have cirrhosis you may live in fear that your condition will deteriorate towards liver failure or malignancy. Liver cancer, as we've seen, usually carries a bleak prognosis and you may need to come to terms with your death. And liver diseases can impose a considerable mental toll, especially as people need to juggle their commitments or feel guilty about the time they spend managing their disease or the condition's impact on their families.

Not surprisingly, many people with liver disease develop psychiatric problems. In one study, almost a quarter of people with chronic liver diseases – including HCV and HBV infection, and NAFLD – also had depression. Excessive alcohol consumption (more than 10 g a day – just over 1 unit) made the depression worse for people with HCV or HBV.[3] Furthermore, everyone with chronic liver disease – and their carers – needs to ensure they get a good night's sleep. Fatigue increased the risk of depression in people with HCV.[3] In people with primary biliary cirrhosis (page 76), fatigue increased the likelihood of anxiety and depression. Fatigued PBC patients also tended to worry excessively.[4]

Don't underestimate depression or anxiety

Sleep disturbances can also be a symptom of depression and anxiety. Depression is more than feeling 'down in the dumps'. It is profound, debilitating mental and physical lethargy, a pervasive sense of worthlessness and intense, deep, unshakable sadness. Similarly, anxiety is more than feeling a little wound up, worried or stressed out. It is intense, sometimes debilitating, fear – even abject terror. If you've never experienced clinical depression or anxiety it's difficult to appreciate how devastating these conditions are.

People with liver disease are especially likely to suffer depression and anxiety. There is the burden of living with a serious disease and interferons (page 33) and hepatic encephalophy (page 16) can trigger depression. Unfortunately, people living with depression or anxiety are often less motivated to stick to their lifestyle regimens and treatments for liver disease. So, they may be more likely to develop complications.

Tips for a good night's sleep

You can take several steps to help you sleep better without resorting to sleeping pills:

- Wind down or relax at the end of the day: don't go to bed while your mind is still racing or pondering problems.
- Try not to take your troubles to bed with you. Brooding on problems makes them seem worse, exacerbates stress, keeps you awake and, because you're tired in the morning, means you are less able to deal with your difficulties. So, try to avoid heavy discussions before bed.
- Don't worry about anything you've forgotten to do. Get up and jot it down (keep a notepad by the bed if it's a persistent problem). This should help you forget about the problem until the morning.
- Go to bed at the same time each night and set your alarm for the same time each morning, including the weekends. This helps re-establish a regular sleep pattern.
- Avoid naps during the day.
- Avoid stimulants, such as caffeine and nicotine, for several hours before bed. Try hot milk instead.
- Don't drink too much just before bed as this can mean regular trips to the bathroom.
- Avoid alcohol. A nightcap can help you fall asleep but as blood levels fall, sleep becomes more fragmented and lighter. Therefore, you may wake repeatedly in the latter part of the night. You should not drink if you have some form of liver disease in any case.
- Don't eat a heavy meal before bedtime.
- Although regular exercise helps you sleep, exercising just before bed can disrupt sleep.
- Use the bed for sex and sleep only. Don't work or watch TV. This means you associate the bed with sleep.
- Make the bed and bedroom as comfortable as possible. If you can, invest in a comfortable mattress, with enough bedclothes, and make sure the room is not too hot, too cold or too bright.
- If you still can't sleep, get up and do something else. Watch the TV or read, nothing too stimulating, until you feel tired. Lying there worrying about not sleeping just keeps you awake.

Putting yourself in control of your problems is one of the best ways to beat anxiety and depression. On the other hand, feeling that your liver disease (or another problem) controls *you* is one of the most common causes of anxiety, depression and stress related to liver disease or life more generally. Nevertheless, some people need additional help. If symptoms markedly affect your daily life, your doctor may suggest antidepressants or drugs to alleviate anxiety (anxiolytics). Don't dismiss drugs out of hand. It's often difficult to overhaul your lifestyle to help control your liver disease in particular or tackle your life problems in general when you're also carrying the burden imposed by depression or anxiety.

While drugs can ease depression and anxiety, they do not cure the problem. But medicines may offer you a window of opportunity to deal with any other issues you face. Many people find that talking to a counsellor helps them find new ways to live with chronic liver disease, tackle problems more generally and, if they face death, put their affairs in order. If you are terminally ill try talking to your spiritual leader, a cancer specialist or hospice, or contact Cancer UK or Macmillan Cancer Support.

Many people also benefit from consulting counsellors and psychotherapists, who use a variety of 'talking therapies' to help you tackle your problems. One widely used approach – cognitive behavioural therapy (CBT) – helps you identify the feelings, thoughts and behaviours associated with liver disease. CBT will then help you question and test those feelings, thoughts, behaviours and

Depression and partners

Depressed people can feel they are living at the bottom of a deep well; even if they can see the light, it seems faint and distant, and they feel there is no way to climb out. Depression can mean that the person simply cannot motivate themselves to seek help or take their medicines as recommended by their doctor. A sympathetic, supportive partner can encourage a depressed or anxious person with liver disease to seek help. But remember that any ladder you offer may seem rickety and unstable. You can help engender the confidence your partner needs to climb out. Emotional support shows you care and so boosts your partner's feeling of self-worth, which can help improve mental health.

beliefs that are unhelpful and unrealistic and replace these with approaches that help you actively address your problems and live a more fulfilled life. In other words, CBT helps you face issues that you have avoided and try out new ways of behaving and reacting, which bolsters your defences against psychological problems, overcomes practical problems and helps improve your control of liver disease. Contact the British Association for Counselling and Psychotherapy or ask your doctor's surgery if they can recommend a local counsellor.

Starting to tackle stress now can help bolster your defences when things get tough. There are several ways you can keep your stress levels down:

- As stress 'first aid', try breathing in deeply through your nose for the count of four; hold your breath for a count of seven; breathe out for a count of eight. Repeat a dozen times.
- Yoga and exercise both seem to improve mood and reduce anxiety. But yoga may improve mood and reduce anxiety more than the same amount of exercise such as walking. (Yoga does not replace all the cardiovascular benefits of exercise.)
- Some people find that massage, aromatherapy, reflexology, acupressure, t'ai chi and meditation alleviate symptoms, such as tiredness and sore muscles, as well as helping them relax.
- Many herbs can help with fatigue and stress, including astragalus and ginseng.
- Consider hypnosis, which can also help with pain, alleviate stress and help you change your behaviour, and overcome harmful habits such as abusing alcohol, comfort eating or smoking. Some people also find that self-hypnosis helps. Numerous DVDs, CDs and books can help you create the 'focused attention' that underpins hypnosis and suggest other ways of relaxation. Contact the British Association of Medical Hypnosis.

The ripples from liver disease

John Donne famously commented that 'no man is an island' – and friends, families and wider social networks are essential for most people to enjoy good health and effectively manage serious diseases, including liver conditions. However, the ripples from any serious disease spread throughout the family. Walking the tightrope between not letting you do anything and allowing you to do too much, as well as their fears for the future, often make life especially difficult for your family.

Your partner shoulders an especially heavy burden. They may fear being alone if you die. They may worry that they could catch the hepatitis virus during sex. They may need to take precautions to prevent the virus spreading around the family. They may face prejudice from neighbours or 'friends' who do not understand the disease. And in some cases, alcohol or drug abuse may have stretched the relationship to breaking point.

Nevertheless, your family's practical and emotional support is invaluable if you are trying to quit smoking or drinking, change your diet and take your medicines as prescribed. Your partner can help you adopt a healthy lifestyle by changing the shopping list or exercising with you. They can ignore bad moods triggered by nicotine or alcohol withdrawal or some treatments for liver disease, boost your motivation when you feel like quitting and can watch for harmful behaviours, such as offering a gentle reminder if you start eating unhealthy food regularly.

Caring for a person with liver disease can be physically demanding and emotionally draining. So, reassure them that they do not need to feel guilty about taking time out for themselves. Carers should try to rest while you are asleep (see the box 'Tips for a good night's sleep' for some suggestions). And carers should be honest with themselves. Partners of people with liver disease may feel angry, guilty or resentful. Don't let them bottle these feelings up: they should talk to you, friends, family or a counsellor.

As these examples show, coming to terms with a diagnosis of liver disease is rarely easy. But you don't need to feel that you're chained to a rock, the disease pecking away at the remnants of your healthy liver. An active, enquiring approach to your health and well-being helps you loosen the shackles of liver disease.

Useful addresses

Action on Smoking and Health (ASH)
First Floor
144–145 Shoreditch High Street
London E1 6JE
Tel.: 020 7739 5902
Website: www.ash.org.uk

Alcohol Concern
Suite B5, West Wing
New City Cloisters
196 Old Street
London EC1V 9FR
Tel.: 020 7566 9800
Website: www.alcoholconcern.org.uk

Alcoholics Anonymous
PO Box 1
Toft Green
York YO1 7NJ
Helpline: 0845 769 7555
Website: www.alcoholics-anonymous.org.uk

Alpha 1 Awareness UK
PO Box 2866
Eastville
Bristol BS5 5EE
Website: www.alpha1awareness.org.uk

Ayurvedic Practitioners Association
23 Green Ridge
Brighton
East Sussex BN1 5LT
Tel.: 01273 500 492
Website: www.apa.uk.com

British Association of Accredited Ayurvedic Practitioners
5 Blenheim Road
North Harrow
Middlesex HA2 7AQ
Tel.: 020 8427 3342
Website: www.britayurpractitioners.com

British Association for Counselling and Psychotherapy
BACP House
15 St John's Business Park
Lutterworth
Leics LE17 4HB
Tel.: 01455 883300
Website: www.bacp.co.uk

British Association of Medical Hypnosis
45 Hyde Park Square
London W2 2JT
Website: www.bamh.org.uk

British Dietetic Association
Fifth Floor, Charles House
148/9 Great Charles Street
Queensway
Birmingham B3 3HT
Tel.: 0121 200 8080
Website: www.bda.uk.com/index.html

British Heart Foundation
Greater London House
180 Hampstead Road
London NW1 7AW
Tel.: 020 7554 0000 (office);
0300 330 3311 (helpline)
Website: www.bhf.org.uk

British Liver Trust
2 Southampton Road
Ringwood
Hants BH24 1HY
Tel.: 01425 481320 (office);
0800 652 7330 (helpline)
Website: www.britishlivertrust.org.
uk

British Porphyria Association
136 Devonshire Road
Durham City DH1 2BL
Helpline: 01474 369231
Website: www.porphyria.org.uk

Cancer Research UK
Angel Building
407 St John Street
London EC1V 4AD
Tel.: 020 7242 0200 (office);
0300 123 1022 (helpline)
Website: www.cancerresearchuk.org

CORE
3 St Andrews Place
London NW1 4LB
(for donations: Freepost LON4268,
London NW1 0YT)
Tel.: 020 7486 0341
Website: www.corecharity.org.uk
Funds research into the entire
range of gut, liver, intestinal and
bowel illnesses.

**Diabetes Research and Wellness
Foundation**
101–102 Northney Marina
Hayling Island
Hants PO11 0NH
Tel.: 023 92 637808
Website: www.drwf.org.uk

Diabetes UK
Macleod House
10 Parkway
London NW1 7AA
Tel.: 020 7424 1000
Website: www.diabetes.org.uk

**General Regulatory Council for
Complementary Therapies**
Box 437, Office 6
Slington House
Rankine Road
Basingstoke
Hants RG24 8PH
Tel.: 0870 3144031
Website: www.grcct.org

Haemochromatosis Society
Hollybush House
Hadley Green Road
Barnet
Herts EN5 5PR
Tel.: 020 8449 1363
Website:www.haemochromatosis.
org.uk

**Health Care and Professions
Council**
Park House
184 Kennington Park Road
London SE11 4BU
Tel.: 0845 300 6184
Website: www.hcpc-uk.org

Hepatitis B Foundation
The Great Barn
Godmersham Park
Canterbury
Kent CT4 7DT
Tel.: 01227 738279 (general);
08000 461911 (helpline)
Website: www.hepb.org.uk

Hepatitis C Trust
27 Crosby Row
London SE1 3YD
Helpline: 0845 223 4424
Website: www.hepctrust.org.uk

Institute for Complementary and Natural Medicine (and British Register of Complementary Practitioners)
Can-Mezzanine
32–36 Loman Street
London SE1 0EH
Tel.: 020 7922 7980
Website: www.icnm.org.uk

Macmillan Cancer Support
89 Albert Embankment
London SE1 7UQ
Helpline: 0808 808 00 00
Website: www.macmillan.org.uk

National Digestive Diseases Information Clearinghouse
Website: http://digestive.niddk.nih.gov

National Health Service advice on giving up smoking
NHS Smoking Helpline: 0800 022 4 332
Website: www.smokefree.nhs.uk

National Organisation for Foetal Alcohol Syndrome
165 Beaufort Park
London NW11 6DA
Tel.: 020 8458 5951
Website: www.nofas-uk.org
NB If searching elsewhere for information about this syndrome, use the international spelling 'Fetal'.

National Osteoporosis Society
Camerton
Bath BA2 0PJ
Helpline: 0845 450 0230 (9 a.m. to 5 p.m., Monday to Friday)
Website: www.nos.org.uk

NHS Organ Donation Register
Tel.: 0300 123 2323 (to join)
Website: www.organdonation.nhs.uk

Primary Sclerosing Cholangitis Support
Website: www.pscsupport.org.uk

Primary Sclerosing Cholangitis Trust
PO Box 267
Southport PR8 1WD
Tel.: 01704 514377
Website: www.psctrust.com

Stroke Association
Stroke Association House
240 City Road
London EC1V 2PR
Tel.: 020 7566 0300 (general); 0303 303 3100 (helpline: 9 a.m. to 5 p.m., Monday to Friday)
Website: www.stroke.org.uk

Wilson's Disease Support Group UK
Website: www.wilsonsdisease.org.uk

References

Introduction

1 Chen TS, Chen PS. The myth of Prometheus and the liver. *Journal of the Royal Society of Medicine* 1994; **87**: 754–5.
2 Sheron N, Hawkey C, Gilmore I. Projections of alcohol deaths? A wake-up call. *Lancet* 2011; **377**: 1297–9.
3 Parkin DM, Boyd L. 4. Cancers attributable to dietary factors in the UK in 2010. *British Journal of Cancer* 2011; **105**: S19–S23.
4 Riley TR, 3rd, Bhatti AM. Preventive strategies in chronic liver disease: Part I. Alcohol, vaccines, toxic medications and supplements, diet and exercise. *American Family Physician* 2001; **64**: 1555–60.

1 Inside a healthy liver

1 Bhatia LS, Curzen NP, Calder PC, Byrne CD. Non-alcoholic fatty liver disease: A new and important cardiovascular risk factor? *European Heart Journal* 2012; **33**: 1190–200.
2 Lefkowitch JH. Anatomy and Function. In: *Sherlock's Diseases of the Liver and Biliary System*. Chichester/Hoboken, NJ: Wiley-Blackwell; 2011, p. 1–19.
3 Wang JF, Chou KC. Molecular modeling of cytochrome P450 and drug metabolism. *Current Drug Metabolism* 2010; **11**: 342–6.
4 Mazze RS, Strock ES, Bergenstal RM, et al. Detection and Treatment of Type 1 Diabetes. In: *Staged Diabetes Management*. Chichester/Hoboken, NJ: Wiley-Blackwell; 2011, p. 41–75.
5 Underwood BA, Siegel H, Weisell RC, Dolinski M. Liver stores of vitamin A in a normal population dying suddenly or rapidly from unnatural causes in New York City. *American Journal of Clinical Nutrition* 1970; **23**: 1037–42.

2 Symptoms of liver disease

1 Seth D, Haber PS, Syn W-K, Diehl AM, Day CP. Pathogenesis of alcohol-induced liver disease: Classical concepts and recent advances. *Journal of Gastroenterology and Hepatology* 2011; **26**: 1089–105.
2 Shepherd J, Jones J, Takeda A, Davidson P, Price A. Adefovir dipivoxil and pegylated interferon alfa-2a for the treatment of chronic hepatitis B: A systematic review and economic evaluation. *Health Technology Assessment* 2006; **10**: iii-iv, xi-xiv, 1–183.
3 Lester BM, Tronick E, Nestler E, et al. Behavioral epigenetics. *Annals of the New York Academy of Sciences* 2011; **1226**: 14–33.
4 Bischoff-Ferrari HA, Willett WC, Orav EJ, et al. A pooled analysis of

vitamin D dose requirements for fracture prevention. *New England Journal of Medicine* 2012; **367**: 40–9.

5   Robison AJ, Nestler EJ. Transcriptional and epigenetic mechanisms of addiction. *Nature Reviews Neuroscience* 2011; **12**: 623–37.

6   Taylor A, Stapley S, Hamilton W. Jaundice in primary care: A cohort study of adults aged >45 years using electronic medical records. *Family Practice* 2011; **29**: 416–20.

7   Riley TR, 3rd, Bhatti AM. Preventive strategies in chronic liver disease: Part II. Cirrhosis. *American Family Physician* 2001; **64**: 1735–40.

3 Testing for liver disease

1   Bhatia LS, Curzen NP, Calder PC, Byrne CD. Non-alcoholic fatty liver disease: A new and important cardiovascular risk factor? *European Heart Journal* 2012; **33**: 1190–200.

2   Lefkowitch JH. Anatomy and Function. In: *Sherlock's Diseases of the Liver and Biliary System*. Chichester/Hoboken, NJ: Wiley-Blackwell; 2011, p. 1–19.

3   Fleming KM, West J, Aithal GP, Fletcher AE. Abnormal liver tests in people aged 75 and above: Prevalence and association with mortality. *Alimentary Pharmacology and Therapeutics* 2011; **34**: 324–34.

4   Schuppan D, Afdhal NH. Liver cirrhosis. *Lancet* 2008; **371**: 838–51.

4 The A to E of viral hepatitis

1   Javier RT, Butel JS. The history of tumor virology. *Cancer Research* 2008; **68**: 7693–706.

2   Shepherd J, Jones J, Takeda A, Davidson P, Price A. Adefovir dipivoxil and pegylated interferon alfa-2a for the treatment of chronic hepatitis B: A systematic review and economic evaluation. *Health Technology Assessment* 2006; **10**: iii-iv, xi-xiv, 1–183.

3   Woolhouse ME, Howey R, Gaunt E, Reilly L, Chase-Topping M, Savill N. Temporal trends in the discovery of human viruses. *Proceedings of the Royal Society B* 2008; **275**: 2111–5.

4   Asselah T, Lada O, Moucari R, Martinot M, Boyer N, Marcellin P. Interferon therapy for chronic hepatitis B. *Clinical Liver Disease* 2007; **11**: 839–49, viii.

5   Sievert W, Altraif I, Razavi HA, et al. A systematic review of hepatitis C virus epidemiology in Asia, Australia and Egypt. *Liver International* 2011; **31**: 61–80.

6   Cornberg M, Razavi HA, Alberti A, et al. A systematic review of hepatitis C virus epidemiology in Europe, Canada and Israel. *Liver International* 2011; **31**: 30–60.

7   Riley TR, 3rd, Bhatti AM. Preventive strategies in chronic liver disease: Part I. Alcohol, vaccines, toxic medications and supplements, diet and exercise. *American Family Physician* 2001; **64**: 1555–60.

8   Gramenzi A, Caputo F, Biselli M, et al. Review article: Alcoholic

liver disease – pathophysiological aspects and risk factors. *Alimentary Pharmacology and Therapeutics* 2006; **24**: 1151–61.

9 Doyle JS, Aspinall E, Liew D, Thompson AJ, Hellard ME. Current and emerging antiviral treatments for hepatitis C infection. *British Journal of Clinical Pharmacology* 2012 Aug 13 [Epub ahead of print].

10 Lok AS, Gardiner DF, Lawitz E, et al. Preliminary study of two antiviral agents for hepatitis C genotype 1. *New England Journal of Medicine* 2012; **366**: 216–24.

11 Afdhal NH, McHutchison JG, Zeuzem S, et al. Hepatitis C pharmacogenetics: State of the art in 2010. *Hepatology* 2011; **53**: 336–45.

12 Ji J, Sundquist K, Sundquist J. A population-based study of hepatitis D virus as potential risk factor for hepatocellular carcinoma. *Journal of the National Cancer Institute* 2012; **104**: 790–2.

13 Hughes SA, Wedemeyer H, Harrison PM. Hepatitis delta virus. *Lancet* 2011; **378**: 73–85.

5 Alcoholic liver disease

1 Geary T, O'Brien P, Ramsay S, Cook B. A national service evaluation of the impact of alcohol on admissions to Scottish intensive care units. *Anaesthesia* 2012; **67**: 1132–37.

2 Parkin DM. 3. Cancers attributable to consumption of alcohol in the UK in 2010. *British Journal of Cancer* 2011; **105**: S14–S18.

3 Parkin DM, Boyd L. 4. Cancers attributable to dietary factors in the UK in 2010. *British Journal of Cancer* 2011; **105**: S19–S23.

4 Seth D, Haber PS, Syn W-K, Diehl AM, Day CP. Pathogenesis of alcohol-induced liver disease: Classical concepts and recent advances. *Journal of Gastroenterology and Hepatology* 2011; **26**: 1089–105.

5 Gramenzi A, Caputo F, Biselli M, et al. Review article: Alcoholic liver disease – pathophysiological aspects and risk factors. *Alimentary Pharmacology and Therapeutics* 2006; **24**. 1151 61.

6 Non-alcoholic liver disease

1 Parkin DM, Boyd L. 8. Cancers attributable to overweight and obesity in the UK in 2010. *British Journal of Cancer* 2011; **105**: S34–S7.

2 Bhatia LS, Curzen NP, Calder PC, Byrne CD. Non-alcoholic fatty liver disease: A new and important cardiovascular risk factor? *European Heart Journal* 2012; **33**: 1190–200.

3 Riley TR, 3rd, Bhatti AM. Preventive strategies in chronic liver disease: Part I. Alcohol, vaccines, toxic medications and supplements, diet and exercise. *American Family Physician* 2001; **64**: 1555–60.

4 Cusi K. Nonalcoholic fatty liver disease in type 2 diabetes mellitus. *Current Opinion in Endocrinology Diabetes and Obesity* 2009; **16**: 141–9.

5 Shetty SN, Mengi S, Vaidya R, Vaidya AD. A study of standardized extracts of *Picrorhiza kurroa* Royle ex Benth in experimental nonalcoholic fatty liver disease. *Journal of Ayurveda and Integrative Medicine* 2010; **1**: 203–10.

6 Starley BQ, Calcagno CJ, Harrison SA. Nonalcoholic fatty liver disease and hepatocellular carcinoma: A weighty connection. *Hepatology* 2010; **51**: 1820–32.

7 Zhou XH, Qiao Q, Zethelius B, et al. Diabetes, prediabetes and cancer mortality. *Diabetologia* 2010; **53**: 1867–76.

8 Erhardt A, Stahl W, Sies H, Lirussi F, Donner A, Haussinger D. Plasma levels of vitamin E and carotenoids are decreased in patients with non-alcoholic steatohepatitis (NASH). *European Journal of Medical Research* 2011; **16**: 76–8.

9 Sanyal AJ, Chalasani N, Kowdley KV, et al. Pioglitazone, vitamin E, or placebo for nonalcoholic steatohepatitis. *New England Journal of Medicine* 2010; **362**: 1675–85.

7 Liver cancer

1 Abdo AA, Hassanain M, AlJumah A, et al. Saudi guidelines for the diagnosis and management of hepatocellular carcinoma: Technical review and practice guidelines. *Annals of Saudi Medicine* 2012; **32**: 174–99.

2 Kuru B, Camlibel M, Dinc S, Gulcelik MA, Gonullu D, Alagol H. Prognostic factors for survival in breast cancer patients who developed distant metastasis subsequent to definitive surgery. *Singapore Medical Journal* 2008; **49**: 904–11.

3 Forner A, Llovet JM, Bruix J. Hepatocellular carcinoma. *Lancet* 2012; **379**: 1245–55.

4 Sherman M, Llovet JM. Smoking, hepatitis B virus infection, and development of hepatocellular carcinoma. *Journal of the National Cancer Institute* 2011; **103**: 1642–3.

5 Tsai JF, Chuang LY, Jeng JE, et al. Betel quid chewing as a risk factor for hepatocellular carcinoma: A case-control study. *British Journal of Cancer* 2001; **84**: 709–13.

6 Zhou XH, Qiao Q, Zethelius B, et al. Diabetes, prediabetes and cancer mortality. *Diabetologia* 2010; **53**: 1867–76.

7 Parkin DM. 3. Cancers attributable to consumption of alcohol in the UK in 2010. *British Journal of Cancer* 2011; **105**: S14–S18.

8 Parkin DM. 2. Tobacco-attributable cancer burden in the UK in 2010. *British Journal of Cancer* 2011; **105**: S6–S13.

9 Trichopoulos D, Bamia C, Lagiou P, et al. Hepatocellular carcinoma risk factors and disease burden in a European cohort: A nested case–control study. *Journal of the National Cancer Institute* 2011; **103**: 1686–95.

10 Turati F, Edefonti V, Talamini R, et al. Family history of liver cancer and hepatocellular carcinoma. *Hepatology* 2012; **55**: 1416–25.

8 Other diseases of the liver

1 Craig DGN, Bates CM, Davidson JS, Martin KG, Hayes PC, Simpson KJ. Staggered overdose pattern and delay to hospital presentation are associated with adverse outcomes following paracetamol-induced hepatotoxicity. *British Journal of Clinical Pharmacology* 2012; **73**: 285–94.

2   Riley TR, 3rd, Bhatti AM. Preventive strategies in chronic liver disease: Part I. Alcohol, vaccines, toxic medications and supplements, diet and exercise. *American Family Physician* 2001; **64**: 1555–60.
3   Bakhai A, Rigney U, Hollis S, Emmas C. Co-administration of statins with cytochrome P450 3A4 inhibitors in a UK primary care population. *Pharmacoepidemiology and Drug Safety* 2012; **21**: 485–93.
4   Lefkowitch JH. Anatomy and Function. In: *Sherlock's Diseases of the Liver and Biliary System*. Chichester/Hoboken, NJ: Wiley-Blackwell; 2011, p. 1–19.

9 Diet and liver disease

1   Riley TR, 3rd, Bhatti AM. Preventive strategies in chronic liver disease: Part II. Cirrhosis. *American Family Physician* 2001; **64**: 1735–40.
2   Anderson JW, Conley SB. Whole Grains and Diabetes. In: *Whole Grains and Health*. Ames, IA: Blackwell Publishing Professional; 2007, p. 29–46.
3   Kromhout D, Yasuda S, Geleijnse JM, Shimokawa H. Fish oil and omega-3 fatty acids in cardiovascular disease: Do they really work? *European Heart Journal* 2012; **33**: 436–43.
4   Masterton GS, Plevris JN, Hayes PC. Review article: Omega-3 fatty acids – a promising novel therapy for non-alcoholic fatty liver disease. *Alimentary Pharmacology and Therapeutics* 2010; **31**: 679–92.
5   Yokoyama M, Origasa H, Matsuzaki M, et al. Effects of eicosapentaenoic acid on major coronary events in hypercholesterolaemic patients (JELIS): A randomised open-label, blinded endpoint analysis. *Lancet* 2007; **369**: 1090–8.
6   Toeller M. Lifestyle Issues: Diet. In: *Textbook of Diabetes*. Chichester/Hoboken, NJ: Wiley-Blackwell; 2010, p. 346–57.
7   Hunter D, Foster M, McArthur JO, Ojha R, Petocz P, Samman S. Evaluation of the micronutrient composition of plant foods produced by organic and conventional agricultural methods. *Critical Reviews in Food Science and Nutrition* 2011; **51**: 571–82.
8   van der Mark M, Brouwer M, Kromhout H, Nijssen P, Huss A, Vermeulen R. Is pesticide use related to Parkinson disease? Some clues to heterogeneity in study results. *Environmental Health Perspectives* 2012; **120**: 340–7.
9   Armstrong LE, Ganio MS, Casa DJ, et al. Mild dehydration affects mood in healthy young women. *Journal of Nutrition* 2012; **142**: 382–8.
10   Ganio MS, Armstrong LE, Casa DJ, et al. Mild dehydration impairs cognitive performance and mood of men. *British Journal of Nutrition* 2011; **106**: 1535–43.
11   Spigt M, Weerkamp N, Troost J, van Schayck CP, Knottnerus JA. A randomized trial on the effects of regular water intake in patients with recurrent headaches. *Family Practice* 2012; **29**: 370–5.

10 Using herbs to cleanse the liver

1   Ernst E. Alternative detox. *British Medical Bulletin* 2012; **101**: 33–8.

2   Askitopoulou H, Ramoutsaki IA, Konsolaki E. Analgesia and anesthesia: Etymology and literary history of related Greek words. *Anesthesia and Analgesia* 2000; **91**: 486–91.

3   Mustafić H, Jabre P, Caussin C, et al. Main air pollutants and myocardial infarction: A systematic review and meta-analysis. *JAMA: Journal of the American Medical Association* 2012; **307**: 713–21.

4   Diette GB, McCormack MC, Hansel NN, Breysse PN, Matsui EC. Environmental issues in managing asthma. *Respiratory Care* 2008; **53**: 602–15; discussion 16–7.

5   van der Mark M, Brouwer M, Kromhout H, Nijssen P, Huss A, Vermeulen R. Is pesticide use related to Parkinson disease? Some clues to heterogeneity in study results. *Environmental Health Perspectives* 2012; **120**: 340–7.

6   Mahaffey KR. Mercury exposure: Medical and public health issues. *Transactions of the American Clinical and Climatological Association* 2005; **116**: 127–53; discussion 53–4.

7   Johansen P, Mulvad G, Pedersen HS, Hansen JC, Riget F. Human accumulation of mercury in Greenland. *Science of the Total Environment* 2007; **377**: 173–8.

8   Kowalski TE, Falestiny M, Furth E, Malet PF. Vitamin A hepatotoxicity: A cautionary note regarding 25,000 IU supplements. *American Journal of Medicine* 1994; **97**: 523–8.

9   Anderson JW, Conley SB. Whole Grains and Diabetes. In: *Whole Grains and Health*. Ames, IA: Blackwell Publishing Professional; 2007, p. 29–46.

10   Riley TR, 3rd, Bhatti AM. Preventive strategies in chronic liver disease: Part I. Alcohol, vaccines, toxic medications and supplements, diet and exercise. *American Family Physician* 2001; **64**: 1555–60.

11   Nemeth E, Bernath J. Biological activities of yarrow species (*Achillea* spp.). *Current Pharmaceutical Design* 2008; **14**: 3151–67.

12   Stegelmeier BL. Pyrrolizidine alkaloid-containing toxic plants (*Senecio, Crotalaria, Cynoglossum, Amsinckia, Heliotropium*, and *Echium* spp.). *The Veterinary Clinics of North America. Food Animal Practice* 2011; **27**: 419–28.

13   Renneberg R. Biotech history: Yew trees, paclitaxel synthesis and fungi. *Biotechnology Journal* 2007; **2**: 1207–9.

14   Girish C, Pradhan SC. Indian herbal medicines in the treatment of liver diseases: Problems and promises. *Fundamental and Clinical Pharmacology* 2012; **26**: 180–9.

15   Manna P, Sinha M, Sil PC. Aqueous extract of *Terminalia arjuna* prevents carbon tetrachloride-induced hepatic and renal disorders. *BMC Complementary and Alternative Medicine* 2006; **6**: 33.

16   Dang SS, Jia XL, Song P, et al. Inhibitory effect of emodin and Astragalus polysaccharide on the replication of HBV. *World Journal of Gastroenterology* 2009; **15**: 5669–73.

17   Shetty SN, Mengi S, Vaidya R, Vaidya AD. A study of standardized extracts of *Picrorhiza kurroa* Royle ex Benth in experimental nonal-

coholic fatty liver disease. *Journal of Ayurveda and Integrative Medicine* 2010; **1**: 203–10.

18   Abenavoli L, Capasso R, Milic N, Capasso F. Milk thistle in liver diseases: Past, present, future. *Phytotherapy Research* 2010; **24**: 1423–32.

19   Fried MW, Navarro VJ, Afdhal N, et al. Effect of silymarin (milk thistle) on liver disease in patients with chronic hepatitis C unsuccessfully treated with interferon therapy: A randomized controlled trial. *JAMA: Journal of the American Medical Association* 2012; **308**: 274–82.

20   Isbrucker RA, Burdock GA. Risk and safety assessment on the consumption of Licorice root (*Glycyrrhiza* sp.), its extract and powder as a food ingredient, with emphasis on the pharmacology and toxicology of glycyrrhizin. *Regulatory Toxicology and Pharmacology* 2006; **46**: 167–92.

21   Hajiaghamohammadi AA, Ziaee A, Samimi R. The efficacy of licorice root extract in decreasing transaminase activities in non-alcoholic fatty liver disease: A randomized controlled clinical trial. *Phytotherapy Research* 2012; **26**: 1381–4.

22   Asl MN, Hosseinzadeh H. Review of pharmacological effects of *Glycyrrhiza* sp. and its bioactive compounds. *Phytotherapy Research* 2008; **22**: 709–24.

23   Xiao J, Ching YP, Liong EC, Nanji AA, Fung ML, Tipoe GL. Garlic-derived S-allylmercaptocysteine is a hepato-protective agent in non-alcoholic fatty liver disease in vivo animal model. *European Journal Nutrition* 2012 Jan 26 [Epub ahead of print].

24   Nwokocha CR, Owu DU, Nwokocha MI, Ufearo CS, Iwuala MOE. Comparative study on the efficacy of *Allium sativum* (garlic) in reducing some heavy metal accumulation in liver of wistar rats. *Food and Chemical Toxicology* 2012; **50**: 222–6.

25   D'Argenio G, Mazzone G, Ribecco MT, et al. Garlic extract attenuating rat liver fibrosis by inhibiting TGF-ß1. *Clinical Nutrition (Edinburgh, Scotland)* 2012 Jul 24 [Epub ahead of print].

26   Ernst E. Risks of herbal medicinal products. *Pharmacoepidemiology and Drug Safety* 2004; **13**: 767–71.

11 Living with liver disease

1   Mills EJ, Wu P, Lockhart I, Thorlund K, Puhan M, Ebbert JO. Comparisons of high-dose and combination nicotine replacement therapy, vareni-cline, and bupropion for smoking cessation: A systematic review and multiple treatment meta-analysis. *Annals of Medicine* 2012; **44**: 588–97.

2   Aubin H-J, Farley A, Lycett D, Lahmek P, Aveyard P. Weight gain in smokers after quitting cigarettes: Meta-analysis. *BMJ* 2012; **345**: e4439.

3   Weinstein AA, Kallman Price J, Stepanova M, et al. Depression in patients with nonalcoholic fatty liver disease and chronic viral hepatitis B and C. *Psychosomatics* 2011; **52**: 127–32.

4   Blackburn P, Freeston M, Baker CR, Jones DE, Newton JL. The role of psychological factors in the fatigue of primary biliary cirrhosis. *Liver International* 2007; **27**: 654–61.

Further reading

Rolande Anderson, *Living with a Problem Drinker*. London: Sheldon Press, 2010.

Roberta Bivins, *Alternative Medicine? A History*. Oxford: Oxford University Press, 2007.

David Conway, *The Magic of Herbs*. London: Jonathan Cape, 1973.

The Doctors' Prescription for Healthy Living, *Healing Hepatitis Naturally*. Topanga, CA: Freedom Press, 2000.

Mark Greener and Christine Craggs-Hinton, *The Diabetes Healing Diet*. London: Sheldon Press, 2012.

Jennifer Harper, *Detox Handbook*. London: Dorling Kindersley, 2002.

Ronald Hutton, *The Stations of the Sun: A History of the Ritual Year in Britain*. Oxford: Oxford University Press, 1996.

Lise Manniche, *An Ancient Egyptian Herbal*. London: British Museum Publications, 1989.

Siddhartha Mukherjee, *The Emperor of All Maladies: A Biography of Cancer*. London: Fourth Estate, 2011.

Julia Tugendhat, *How to Approach Death*. London: Sheldon Press, 2007.

Andrew Weil, *Health and Healing: The Philosophy of Integrative Medicine*. London: Warner Books, 1996.

Andrew Weil, *Spontaneous Healing: How to Discover and Enhance Your Body's Natural Ability to Maintain and Heal Itself*. London: Warner Books, 1997.

Index

aflatoxin 4, 32, 61–2
alcohol viii, ix, 3, 4, 7, 11, 13, 15, 17–18, 24–5, 36–7, 41–51, 53, 62–4, 69–72, 75, 81, 95, 98, 100, 105–6, 113, 117–18, 120–1
alpha-1 antitrypsin deficiency 70, 74–5
anaemia 19, 39, 46, 73
antivirals 33–4, 37–9
anxiety 16, 36, 48, 97, 109, 114, 117–20; see also mental changes
ascites 14, 17–19, 27, 64, 73
autoimmune disease, and hepatitis viii, 18, 22, 70, 76

B vitamins see vitamin B
bile 2, 5, 17–18, 24, 73, 76–7, 96, 106; duct 18, 22–3, 25, 60–1, 68, 76–7; stones see gallstones
bilirubin 13, 17–18, 25–6, 77
biopsy 23–4, 54, 65–6
bleeding problems 10, 14–17, 19–20, 27, 60, 73–4
blood 9, 15; clotting see bleeding problems; vomiting 12, 19
bones, brittle and broken see osteoporosis

cancer: general 18–19, 20, 25–6, 33, 42, 52, 56, 59–60, 63, 65, 87, 94, 103, 106, 110, 113–14; liver see liver cancer
Child–Pugh score 26–7, 67–8, 106
Chinese medicine, traditional 1, 107–8, 111–12
cholesterol 8–9, 53, 56, 77–80, 84–6, 90, 93, 96
cirrhosis viii, ix, 11, 12–17, 32, 35–7, 40, 44, 46, 53, 61, 64, 66, 70, 76, 83, 87, 105–6, 117
coagulation see blood clotting
cognitive behavioural therapy 119–20
complementary therapy 82, 97, 99–112, 119–20; see also herbs, hypnosis
counselling 48, 50–1, 119–120
cryptogenic liver disease 70
cytochromes see liver enzymes

deaths see liver disease, deaths from
depression 16, 33, 36–7, 48–9, 51, 107, 111; see also mental changes
detox ix, 82, 90, 92, 97–9, 100–2; see also herbs

diabetes viii, 22, 52, 54, 56–8, 62, 78, 82, 84, 87–8, 90–1, 94, 98, 103, 117–20
diet, healthy 11, 45, 54–6, 75, 82–98, 100, 113
dieting, as way of losing weight 55–7, 84, 90, 92–7, 120
drug: abuse ix, 17, 29–31, 34–5, 40, 115, 121; interactions 5, 79–80, 111–12

emphysema 2, 74–5
energy, role of liver in 7
exercise 52, 54–5, 75, 82, 85, 96–7, 115, 118, 120

faeces: bloody 19, 64; colour of 12, 17–18, 40, 64–5, 74, 77
fat: in blood see cholesterol, triglycerides; in the body see obesity and overweight; in diet 7–8, 56, 82, 84–5, 88, 94–5
fatigue 12, 14, 19, 33, 36, 39–40, 58, 73, 81, 97, 102, 104, 117, 119–20
fatty liver disease see steatosis
fibre 78, 90–4
fibrosis, liver 12, 23, 53, 104, 107–9
fish 16, 56, 85–90
free radicals 45, 55–6, 82, 85, 91, 106, 108
fruit 30, 41, 75, 79, 82, 86, 90–2, 94, 97, 116

gall bladder 1–2, 23, 70, 96, 101, 103, 105
gallstones 18, 77–8, 94, 96, 99, 101
garlic 108–9, 111
glucose 7, 57–8

headache 39, 97–8, 100, 102, 109
haem viii, 9, 71; see also porphyrins
haemochromatosis 70, 72
haemophilia 30, 31, 34
heart disease 9, 26, 52, 57, 79, 82–4, 88, 94, 101, 113–14
hepatic encephalopathy see mental changes
hepatitis viii, 11, 28, 32, 40, 44, 58, 88, 99, 104–6; A virus (HAV) 28–30, 39, 108; B virus (HBV) 14, 28, 30–5, 39, 61–4, 69, 104, 108, 117; C virus (HCV) 11, 13, 21, 31, 32–3, 35–9, 44, 61–4, 72, 81, 107–8, 117; D virus (HDV) 39–40; E virus (HEV) 40–1

hepatitis viruses viii, ix, 11, 17–18, 21–2, 64, 69, 105, 107; tests for *see* viral load; *see also individual viruses*
hepatocellular carcinoma *see* liver cancer
hepatocyte 3, 6, 16, 28, 33, 45, 60, 80, 106
herbs ix, 6, 80, 97, 99–112, 120
hormones 15, 17, 46, 78, 84, 100–1
hypnosis 116, 120

insomnia *see* sleep problems
interferon 33, 37–9, 40, 69, 107, 117
itching 12–14, 39, 65, 77, 81

jaundice viii, 12, 14, 17–18, 23, 28–9, 32, 40, 65, 73–4, 77, 81, 104–5

kava kava 109–11
kidney disease 9, 17, 25, 34, 57, 101, 109

liquorice 108–9
liver: cancer viii, ix, 1, 17, 23–4, 32, 35, 36, 40, 54, 59–69, 117; cell *see* hepatocyte; enzymes 5–6, 24–6, 33, 49, 55, 58, 79–81, 102, 106–8, 111; failure *see* liver disease, end-stage; flushes and cleanses 100–2; function tests 24–6, 33, 40, 54–5, 65, 81; healthy 1–10; inflammation of *see* hepatitis; location in the body 2; regeneration of vii, 20; scarring *see* cirrhosis; tonics ix, 99–112; transplant 20, 66–7, 69, 76–7, 110; tumours, benign 59–60
liver disease: deaths from vii, 20, 25, 32, 39, 42, 59–61, 66–7, 117, 119; end-stage 20, 53, 66–7, 70, 73–7, 110, 117; imaging for 22–3, 65–6; symptoms of viii, 11, 14, 21, 29, 36, 64–5; *see also* individual symptoms
lymph 4–5

medicines, and liver damage 7, 70–1, 80–1
mental changes 11, 16, 27, 33, 107, 117–20
milk thistle 49, 99, 105–7, 111

non-alcoholic fatty liver disease (NAFLD) 26, 52–8, 62, 82, 84, 87, 90–1, 94, 102, 105, 108, 117
non-alcoholic steatohepatitis (NASH) *see* non-alcoholic fatty liver disease
nuts 56, 74, 85–6, 89, 91–4

obesity and overweight 8, 18, 44, 52–3, 62–3, 78, 82, 94–6, 116

oedema 17, 73
oils 56, 85, 86, 89–90
osteoporosis 15–17, 73, 87

paracetamol 6, 70, 79, 81, 105, 108, 111
Parkinson's disease 93, 101
pesticides 93, 100–1
pollution 56, 75, 100–1
porphyrins viii, 9, 70–2
portal hypertension 15, 17, 19, 77
pregnancy 31, 34, 40–1, 46, 76
primary biliary cirrhosis 22, 70, 76, 117
primary sclerosing cholangitis 70, 77
Prometheus vii, 12
protein 8, 16, 25, 87, 94, 104, 106

St John's wort 6, 79, 111
salt 19, 82–4, 92, 95
seeds 56, 85, 87, 89–94
sex ix, 12, 30–1, 34, 36, 40, 118, 121
silymarin *see* milk thistle
sleep problems 16, 48, 109–10, 114, 117–18
smoking viii, 11, 56, 63, 69, 74, 75, 100, 113–16, 118, 120–1
spider naevi 12, 14
spleen 15, 17, 101
steatosis 8, 23, 44, 45, 52–4, 58, 88, 105, 108; *see also* non-alcoholic fatty liver disease
stress 47, 51, 76, 115–20
strokes 9, 52, 57, 68, 79, 83–4, 113
surgery, risks 24, 27

tiredness *see* fatigue
toxins 3, 16, 24, 53, 70, 76, 80, 90, 97, 100–6, 108–9, 114
triglycerides 8, 53, 78, 88

urine, colour of viii, 12, 17–18, 40, 57, 65, 70–1

vaccination 30, 31, 34–5, 39
varices 15, 19–20
vegetables 55, 56, 74, 82, 85, 89–92, 97
viral load 21, 33, 34, 37
viruses *see* hepatitis viruses
vitamins: A 9, 45, 55, 85, 102; B 45–6, 85, 91; C 45; D 15, 85; E 45, 55–6, 58, 85, 91

weight loss, unexplained 12, 14, 58, 65, 81
Wilson's disease 70, 73–4, 101